E

"**I**f you have a loved one suffering the ravages of dementia of any kind, you need this heartfelt book from Joni Wyatt. It's compelling, vulnerable and, most of all, comforting."

— **Dr. Les Parrott,** #1 New York Times
bestselling author of *Love Like That*

"**Y**ou may not need this book right now, but someday you might, and you will want to have it near. Had Joni's book been available to my own family as our mother, Margaret, went through the valley of Alzheimer's, we would have been better prepared. I commend these writings to you and know you will be encouraged by the practical advice, Scriptural truth, and genuine celebration of both tears and laughter. Thank you, Joni, for allowing us the privilege of peeking into these personal family times. You have helped us to be better children and caregivers."

— **Dr. Bob Broadbooks,** USA/Canada
Regional Director of Church of the Nazarene

"Joni has written from the heart . . . to the heart of those who suffer most when Alzheimer's comes to a family—the caregivers. Hold the promises of this book close, even when those you love most push you away as you're trying to help. The road you are walking may be the hardest calling in life, but Joni's insights, and the promises of the Scripture will make your struggle easier to understand."

— **Dr. Roger Parrott,** President of Belhaven University

"A powerful, soul-lifting read. Absolutely brilliant work—so authentic, poignant, observant, filled with compassion and deft touches of humor. The core truth, you captured it superbly! The absence of time. Sounds like the beginning of eternity to me."

— **Misty L. Calhoun**

ACKNOWLEDGEMENTS

The journey with Dad, and Mom, through the mire, sludge and heartache of Alzheimer's disease was not taken by me alone. I am incredibly grateful for, and indebted to:

- Every person from each doctor's office, hospital, and living facility. Those who physically cared for my parents and treated them with dignity.
- Everyone who visited from near and far, sang, sent letters, called and prayed, giving emotional and spiritual care to my parents.
- My family, and extended family, all of you, who have McCleery in your name, or in your blood!
- Misty, you kept me sane, my lifelong friend. I love you!
- Especially thankful for Deb Geffert. You are an angel! Love You!
- Amy Hollingsworth, you gave us the greatest gift in the journey—our "last good night" with Mom. We will cherish it the rest of our days. I love you dearly!

McKenna, McCleery, and McLane, my darling children. Thank you, thank you, thank you for the unending kindness, love, and care you gave Gram and Papa! You made their final days infinitely more bearable. I love you each "the most!"

I could never formulate the words, expressions, or depth of meaning in a "thank you" to my dearest, sweetest, most patient, resilient, and loving husband, Doug. I love you. Always.

I am, most of all, humbly grateful to my Jesus . . .
my Savior, my Friend, my Confidant, and my Strength.
I am in awe of Your never-ending junctures.

DEDICATION

I dedicate this work to you, the caregiver.

43 JUNCTURES *with Jesus*

43 JUNCTURES *with Jesus*

Encouragement for Caregivers

JONI WYATT

EQUIP PRESS

Colorado Springs

43 JUNCTURES with Jesus

Published by Equip Press, Colorado Springs, CO

First Edition: 2018
43 Junctures with Jesus / Joni Wyatt
Paperback ISBN: 978-1-946453-52-5
eBook ISBN: 978-1-946453-51-8

EQUIP PRESS

Colorado Springs

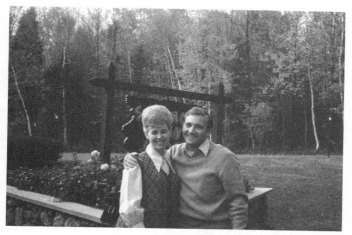

MEET MY PARENTS

I would like to introduce you to a couple who are rare, if not extinct, in this world. They are of another time and another era.

Their focus and driving force in life was to glorify God. Sounds simple enough, yet my parents epitomized the ideal of what it means to serve as, "pastor and wife."

Both of my parents were not raised in a Christian home.

My mom, Joan, was born in Missouri in 1930 and began attending church at age nine or ten, because her father had made a deal with God. The deal was: "You save my daughter, I'll go to church." Mom had been near death from an appendix operation. Soon after they began attending, she asked Jesus into her heart.

Mom thought the greatest calling a woman could have was to be a pastor's wife.

Dad, Lee (Roy), was born in 1935 and raised on a farm in Oklahoma by an abusive, alcoholic father, and sweet, compliant mother. At age seventeen, Dad's family went to church, and all were radically saved, including his father, my grandfather.

Dad thought the greatest calling a man could have was to be a pastor.

They married in 1959. For nearly fifty years they served God, pastored, and ministered wherever He sent them—all over this country! They were a powerhouse for Christ! Everything they did was for God and the church.

They visited the sick, lonely, and brokenhearted. They shared meals, thousands of meals, with folks. They wrote cards, made phone calls, and checked on people. They taught Sunday school, children's church, ladies' programs, men's programs, VBS, directed camps and retreats, etc., etc.

But what they did *most* of all was LOVE people, just like Jesus did. If you knew the McCleerys, then you were LOVED by the McCleerys!

It was the breath in their lungs. And, they did it incredibly well! They are deeply loved and greatly remembered by all whom were touched by them.

Our arrival in heaven will reveal the true far-reaching effects their ministry has had.

Lee and Joan McCleery were my parents. They both had Alzheimer's disease.

I consider it my greatest privilege to have had the opportunity to honor them during the last five years of their lives.

INTRODUCTION

The journey through dementia and the family of diseases it represents is unlike anything you could imagine. It is one wild ride!

It begins slowly and subtly. You notice some lapses in your loved one's cognition, but easily brush them aside, attributing them to the inevitability of advancing age. For instance, there was a time when my father was sure he saw an Australian dingo in his backyard in Kansas. Or, the time he "remembered" the frigid air of Mt. Everest as he climbed. *Kinda funny. He's just getting older.* That's what we told ourselves.

The disease progresses. Everyday living becomes more difficult. Bills don't get paid. The power company calls—the power is about to be turned off. *That's* not *Dad, he was meticulous with his money. Hmmmmm, I will have to help a bit, he's just getting older.* That's what we told ourselves.

It continually progresses. More concerning events begin to happen. Poor choices are made. Dad put every gun he owned in the trunk of the car (to keep them safe) while driving to Minnesota. *Worrisome. Why would he do that? We just need to explain to him why that's not a good idea. He will understand.* That's what we told ourselves.

The downward spiral seems to accelerate. Dad would walk away and could disappear in an instant. He didn't know where he was. *This was truly frightening. There is something serious happening here.* We knew we had to intervene.

It is extremely difficult to accept what is happening. It is extremely difficult to walk through. Every day brings new challenges.

But, there are some things you can be sure of:

- God will be with you.
- There is tremendous help from the medical field, doctors, nurses, facilities, and support.
- You are not alone.

I have been where you are finding yourself now. I have written these experiences to give you confidence, courage, help, and hope as you journey through this disease with your loved one.

As you read through them, I have arranged these encounters in chronological order. When we began caring for my parents, they moved to North Dakota where we were living at the time. We moved to Kansas about a year into the journey.

This is the progression of facilities in Kansas where they each had lived:

- Both began in an assisted living facility, Mom on one side, Dad in the locked unit.

- Dad became violent, necessitating his move to a geriatric psychiatric facility, where they regulated his medications to keep him subdued.
- Next, Dad went to a nursing home about an hour from where we lived.
- From there he was moved to a nursing facility right next door to the assisted living facility where Mom was.
- Mom eventually moved over to be in the same place as Dad was. Again, he was in a locked unit; she was on the other side.
- They both left this world from this last place to make their way to their eternal home, twenty months apart from each other.

One thing to note: Alzheimer's manifests itself differently in each person. There are definite similarities, such as the memory loss, but each case of Alzheimer's is uniquely different to the person with the disease. Keep that in mind as you walk through it. This was quite true with my parents:

- Dad wandered; Mom didn't
- Dad lost the ability to talk; Mom didn't
- Dad forgot all of us; Mom didn't
- Dad got violent; Mom didn't

- Mom undermined our decisions; Dad didn't
- Mom minimized reality; Dad wasn't aware of reality
- Mom was overly emotional; Dad wasn't
- Mom always wondered, "Why?"; Dad didn't

Each day, each moment, each journey, with each person, is unique. Unique.

I sincerely pray for God's sustaining power and presence as you daily have a *Juncture with Jesus.*

THE BEGINNING

I knew something wasn't right.

My husband, children, and I were visiting my parents for a few days and on our way to their favorite barbeque restaurant in Overland Park, Kansas. I hadn't lived in Kansas for many years, and I knew the way—it was a very familiar route and we ate there anytime we were in town. We all knew the way. Strangely, Dad kept asking what road to take and which way to turn. "Do I turn left at the next light?" "No, Dad, you turn right." I could tell he was nervous and unsure about getting there. *Why was he asking where to turn?* He didn't know where the restaurant was. *How could that be?* Mom was irritated and put out at his hesitations and questioning, so she responded with a long, high-pitched, "Honeeeey, you *know* where it is!" It was extremely unsettling and alarming for me. I knew something was definitely wrong. Very, very wrong.

It was on that night, in that car ride and in those tension-filled moments, with the dawning realization that something was really wrong, I began a journey with my parents. A journey I had never foreseen, never imagined, and something I knew absolutely nothing about. It was a sojourn forever impacted by Alzheimer's disease. As my family and I plunged forward, God reminded me in Hebrews 13, "I will never leave you, never will I forsake you."

I have now completed the journey. It is over. For five years, my husband, my children, and I daily walked with my father and mother, who BOTH were afflicted with the disease. The experience was a tumultuous mixture of highs and lows, joys and sorrows. But, I believe we each are better for the journey. We lived and learned firsthand to hang on (some days by our fingertips!) to Jesus. To His grace, wisdom, comfort, and strength. He was true to His word, He never left us.

I am attempting to share some experiences, thoughts, and Scriptures that gave me the ability to face whatever the new day held.

Some junctures with Jesus.

I pray God's peace, and His strength, as you are on this journey now . . .

CONTENTS

JUNCTURE ONE

I See You

*"Open my eyes that I may see wonderful things
in your law."*
— (PSALM 119:18, NIV)

Perfectly "normal." At the beginning, that is what dementia looks like. To look at someone suffering, you cannot distinguish the debilitating disease. The person may still be well-groomed, clothed properly, and have eyes that focus and respond. All appearances concealing well the disease lurking inside. Even after a diagnosis, it can be quite difficult to grasp the severity and gravity of the prognosis.

It was hard to detect in Dad. He looked "normal." Generally, he acted "normal," and mostly his conversations were "normal." For Mom, having known him and having lived a life with him for fifty years, it was not "normal." But to reconcile a life-threatening disease that wasn't visible was excruciating. It "looked" like mental illness. To someone with pre-conceived stereotypes of mental illness, this was a terrible blow. Therefore, she hid it and dealt with the descent downhill, privately and painfully, choosing not to see or acknowledge it. As did many others. It is infinitely better to recognize and address the disease.

The Zulu people of South Africa have a traditional greeting, given in two parts. When two people meet, they look intentionally, meaningfully into each other's eyes:

The first person says, "Sikhona" (I am here to be seen). Alzheimer's says, "I desperately need you to recognize me."

The second person replies, "Sawubona" (I see you). Our response, "I recognize and will advocate on your behalf."

How desperately the Alzheimer's sufferer needs to be truly seen, not to be explained away.

With God's strength and courage, you, the caregiver, can look and genuinely "see" your loved one. If you "see" sooner rather than later, your journey with dementia will be much easier for them. And for you.

Sawubona, I see you.

Dear Jesus, thank you that you see us. Give us the conviction to see with your eyes and the strength for what lies ahead.

Reflections:

_____
_____
_____
_____
_____

JUNCTURE TWO

Joyride

"When my worry is great within me, your comfort
brings joy to my soul."
— (Psalm 94:19, NLV)

There is much to lament during the course of Alzheimer's disease. The loss of memory, the decline in health, the changes in personality. But if you adjust your lenses a bit, you are able to find joy.

North Dakota has a rugged, nearly unspoiled beauty. It has expansive blue skies, rolling grasslands, and roaming buffalo. It was on a postcard-worthy day that we decided to take Dad and the kids bike riding. We loaded the bikes, kids, and Dad up, then headed to the nearby state park. This state park was the former home of an old military fort, chosen for its rather hilly terrain in the generally flat prairies. We parked close to the top of a hill and unloaded: bikes, kids, and Dad.

Ohhhh, boy!

Dad, in his state of mind, had no thought of anything except the thrill of riding the bike. He hopped on and catapulted past us, down the hill, down the road, dangerously fast, and really close to any vehicles on the pavement. He didn't look sideways, he didn't look back, he just flew away! I can only imagine the glorious feeling of gliding down that hill, with the fresh air and sunshine as your companions and not a care in the world. For us it was several minutes of frightful anxiety until we caught up with him and knew he was safe. For Dad it was exhilarating. He was beaming, full of life and energy! For us, it was stressful and scary. For Dad it was total freedom. For us it was nerve wracking and worrisome. For Dad it was a fantastic joyride!

Thank you, Jesus, that in the midst of this difficult terrain, you can so simply and beautifully remind us of your joy! Living every day with you is a joyride as I trust in your strength to carry me through!

Reflections:

_____
_____
_____
_____

Sugar Shack

*"For God is not a God of disorder but of peace—as
in all the congregations of the Lord's people."*
— (1 COR. 14:33, NIV)

Folks with dementia lose sight of reality. In various
degrees, reasoning and common sense exit their daily
living. It can be gradual—a statement or action appears that
isn't quite "normal." Or there can be a pronounced moment
in which it is glaringly obvious that the end has come for
certain activities. This end must occur for everyone's well-
being and safety.

Big Sunday dinners, Christmas, Easter, and birthdays.
Mother loved to entertain. Family coming to visit, the
grandkids, or even if it was just Tuesday or Wednesday, she
was able to make any day a holiday. As a child and teenager,
dinner was cooked, plated, and served promptly every

evening at five o'clock. That was a sacred time in our home, and we all knew never to be late! The best part was that each and every meal ended with a freshly baked, yummy dessert!

As Alzheimer's invaded her mind, my mom continued to entertain—just not as often, or elaborately. Arthritis and osteoporosis had also ganged up on her and made it difficult physically. Of all the components of the meal to prepare, her ultimate favorite and highlight was dessert. Although she made the best meatloaf (the secret was sugar in the recipe), her heart was always with dessert, because sugar was her special friend. Oh, how she loved sweets! And how she loved to provide them for us when we were coming over for dinner!

It was one event, one moment, and one last hurrah when we all knew her days of entertaining were over. She had invited my little family for dinner. When we arrived the meal was artfully displayed on the kitchen island. It consisted of: meatloaf (filled with sugar), rolls, cookies, pie, cake, cream cheese brownies, and more cookies. Our eyes were wide with astonishment, jaws dropped, and drooling. Each of us, (including the children), knew this was not in touch with reality. It may sound like a meal in paradise, but it was too much, unbalanced, and definitely unhealthy. It was the last "meal" she prepared (she didn't realize it). Mother always had a flair for the extravagant. And what a spectacular finish!

Jesus, please give me the proper perspective on the events happening. Remind me that you are the One who restores order and peace.

Reflections:

_____

_____

_____

_____

_____

JUNCTURE FOUR

So Convenient

"You gave life and gracious love to me; your
providential care has preserved my spirit."
— (JOB 10:12, ISV)

During the progression of Alzheimer's, there is a period
of time when many routine life functions are still
possible—theoretically. Reality is something altogether
different and difficult.

We had just enjoyed a meal out together. My husband,
our three children, and myself. These times were becoming
rare in the days of caring for my folks.

As we exited the restaurant, I noticed a car across the
parking lot that seemed out of place. There were several
stores in a row with no delineation between the sidewalk
and parking lot. It was all one level. A newer type of strip
mall (which most certainly helps folks with mobility issues).
The car I observed was parked completely on the sidewalk,

parallel to the side of a discount store, within inches of the entrance door. Parallel lengthwise, inches from the door. As I looked, a knot began to form in my stomach as I recognized the car. Yes, it was my parents' vehicle. My dad had parked the car parallel to the store, on the sidewalk, inches from the entrance.

We hurried over and entered the store. Oh, how surprised and happy Mom and Dad were to see us! Thankfully, they had just finished their shopping and were leaving. We escorted them out to the car —the car parked in the most convenient spot in the lot! And they blissfully drove off. We made sure they got home safely. The "convenient spot" was a catalyst to the inevitability of Dad no longer driving.

> *Jesus, thank you for your Divine intervention. I marvel at your orchestration of the details when I'm lost in the middle of it. With you, there is no delineation of "sidewalk" and "parking lot." You cover it all. I rest in that.*

Reflections:

_____

_____

_____

_____

JUNCTURE FIVE

A Hiding Place

"You are my hiding place—
You will protect me from distress.
You surround me with songs of deliverance."
— (Ps. 32:7, TLV)

Alzheimer's gives some folks the compulsion to place items in secret places for safekeeping. There are two major challenges with this behavior: 1.) Choosing reasonable hiding places, and 2.) Remembering where the items are located.

Carter was his first. It was a '57 Chevy—two tone, hardtop, India Ivory, Canyon Coral. He had purchased the classic vehicle from the original owner, Mrs. Carter, the widow of his hometown's pharmacist. It was a project perfectly suited for Dad. It required meticulous precision, and he spent weeks and months lovingly restoring the beauty. It was perfection.

A two-tone, Tropical-Turquoise, India-Ivory Bel Air was the '55 model Dad acquired next. He again meticulously, piece by piece, took it apart and began repairing, replacing, and repainting each part. There were hundreds of parts, maybe more. Small parts, large ones, screws, nuts, bolts, bits of metal, rubber, and cloth. As time progressed, so did Alzheimer's and the difficulty in re-assembling the vehicle. Dad couldn't do it. He wanted to, he tried to, but it became too difficult.

God graciously sent a generous friend willing to buy the car in pieces. We began putting parts in boxes for him. That's when we discovered we were on a treasure hunt. There were car parts in virtually every drawer, box, shelf, and container in the garage. There were car parts in the basement, in the laundry room, in the living room, and bedroom. Parts in drawers, parts in closets, parts in cabinets, and many more "special" spots. I believe Dad, in his confusion, knew these pieces of the car needed to be kept safe and protected, so he found secure locations to store them. The little turquoise-colored bit of metal I discovered in a porcelain teapot and tea cup after our friend had taken the car were reminders of Dad, in his illness, protecting that which was treasured by him.

Jesus, thank you that you are our hiding place.
When all the world seems senseless, you are here for
our protection, no matter where we find ourselves.

Reflections:

_____

_____

_____

_____

_____

JUNCTURE SIX

It's All in the Wrist

"He has [graciously] remembered His
lovingkindness and His faithfulness to the house of
Israel; All the ends of the earth have witnessed the
salvation of our God."
— (Ps. 98:3, AMP)

"Remember your word to your servant, for you
have given me hope."
— (Ps 119:49, NIV)

Most likely, during the course of your experience caring for someone with Alzheimer's disease, you will find yourself in an unusual, unlikely, uncomfortable, or unfamiliar situation. But in those unrelenting moments, hours, and days, there can be unrivaled assurance. God is, and will be, with you unwaveringly, unequivocally, unconditionally, and unbelievably!

Christmas 1976—the year our nation celebrated two hundred years—I received a fantastic gift: a ping-pong table. I wanted one, not really believing it would materialize—but there it was! It was such a wonderful surprise, a gift everyone could use, but it was specifically given to me! We played and played and played ping-pong on that table. We all enjoyed it greatly. But Dad, I believe, enjoyed it most of all.

He was a competitor. When Dad began a game, any game, of any skill level, he was determined to win. Ping-pong was no exception. He watched and studied the Olympic ping-pong matches, teams, and coaches. He read articles and tips on how to improve his serve, and his return. He memorized the rules of the game. He was a fierce opponent.

"It's all in the wrist." That was the one paramount admonition. If you flick your wrist in just the right way, you can spin the ball causing your opponent to either not return it, or it flies off the table wildly. "It's all in the wrist." He was excellent at flicking his wrist and spinning that ball.

Decades later we found ourselves in a psychiatric ward. My brilliant, highly educated father was locked in a hospital psych ward. In my head I understood it was the safest, best, and only option for him to be during a short-term transition. But my eyes and heart were wracked with pain at the reality. It was unbelievably difficult.

Then God reminded me He was there.

It was the ping-pong table. They had one in the middle of the common area in the psych unit. Dad was wandering in circles; we were visiting, following him, trying to talk to him and get him to sit for a moment. He stopped at the ping-pong table. He picked up the paddle, looked it over, turned it this way and that. A wonderful young man working that evening asked him if he wanted to play. Dad agreed. I was skeptical and intrigued. How could he play? He can't form a complete sentence or stand still for thirty seconds.

The young man hit the ball to my father. As that ball came sailing over the net, Dad transformed. He planted his feet just so, he held his paddle like an Olympic champ, he trained his eyes on that ball, and waited. "It's all in the wrist." When it arrived, he flicked his wrist and sent it spinning back to the young man who was unable to return it! Incredible! Then he served, and flicked his wrist again, and again, and again. We all watched amazed! For me it was a reminder of God's unending presence in every situation—and a glimpse of Dad from years ago. All of that in the locked psych ward of the hospital.

Thank you, Jesus, for your undeserving love, your unfathomable presence, and your unending peace. Thank you that I know you have remembered me, wherever I am.

Reflections:

_____

_____

_____

_____

_____

JUNCTURE SEVEN

There's No Place like Home

"And this righteousness will bring peace. Yes, it will bring quietness and confidence forever. My people will live in safety, quietly at home. They will be at rest."

— (ISA. 32:17–18, NLT)

Home. This is difficult for those with Alzheimer's. They may have moments in which they want to "go home." Even if they are in the home they have lived in for most of their life. Or they may be confused and lost in the new surroundings in which they find themselves and, again, want to go home. One of the most helpful things I learned while navigating this wretched disease was that "home" isn't necessarily a place. It is a feeling. (Lightbulb moment!)

What feelings does the word "home" conjure up for you? Safety? Security? Comfort? Peace? Warmth and love? Yes, to all of the above. For most of us, "home" overwhelms us with a sense of being cared for, loved, comforted, and looked after. We can readily transport ourselves back to the time in life when all was simple and good, our needs were met, and we had few worries. Those feelings can envelop us fairly easily, wherever we may be.

On several occasions Dad asked, or attempted, to go "home." Home to Dad meant the farm in Oklahoma—the windswept wheat fields where he was raised. Once, while we were still in North Dakota, he decided to "go home" during a blizzard. It was seventeen degrees below zero outside, and he had left the condo with a light jacket on, telling my mother he was "going home." She was hysterical. She convinced him to come back inside and called us. We prayed that we could make it over there, since there was a blizzard happening, and that Dad wouldn't leave again before we got there. God was gracious and gave us safe passage. When we arrived, Dad told us that he had dropped some books off to "Mrs. Riddle" (Mom, before she married dad), and he was heading "home." He was not sure why she was so adamant about his staying. It was a long, emotional night. Dad needed some reassurance and a measure of comfort. He was terribly confused and just wanted to "go home." The hysterics of my mother and the barrage of information and facts about reality from us were overwhelming for him. With the morning came better spirits, less confusion, and the idea of "going home" was forgotten until another day.

If we had known to address the issue as a feeling, instead of a place, my husband and I could have talked about Dad's family, the farm, and that it might not be good to go "home" in such weather. And, just maybe, our long night would have been a little shorter.

Jesus, please give us wisdom to know how to lovingly address these difficult moments. Thank you that we know our ultimate safety, peace, comfort, and rest will be found with you in our heavenly home.

Reflections:

_____

_____

_____

_____

_____

JUNCTURE EIGHT

Seeing with Different Eyes

> *"But my **eyes** are fixed on you, Sovereign Lord; in*
> *you I take refuge . . ."*
> — *(Ps.141:8, NIV)*

Alzheimer's dementia is a disease. It affects the brain. It changes how information gets from one part of the brain to another. It affects how one views the world—it is a skewed view or not-quite-reality perception.

We were moving from North Dakota to Kansas. One of the most difficult events for folks with Alzheimer's is to change surroundings. My parents had moved up to North Dakota just two years earlier to be near us. It was very hard on them, especially for Dad. He had declined rapidly. Now we were moving them again. We were flying my parents to Kansas to get them settled in to an assisted living facility a few weeks prior to our arrival. I was very nervous in the airport—my father had become increasingly unpredictable. He was prone to wander off.

My husband and I were trying to keep him occupied (i.e., corralled and inconspicuous) before we boarded the plane. The Bismarck airport is an up-to-date, international airport in a city of approximately fifty thousand people. There are exactly two gates—total. Not much chance of blending in with the crowd. The travelers in the tiny terminal were doing whatever it is they do while waiting to board. Several feet from us a young man and woman had a large, hiking-type of backpack they were adjusting. Both of them were kneeling on either side of the bag securing flaps and tying it snugly. Dad glanced over, saw them kneeling and announced, "they're praying." Then, without hesitation, he knelt. And he began to pray. He prayed in his deep, booming, pastoral voice that was as natural to him as breathing. He was completely unaware, unconcerned, and unhindered by his surroundings. He had no inkling of the "real" situation going on around him. He just saw the invitation to pray and took it! My dear, wonderful husband who loved and honored my father, immediately knelt beside him and joined him in lifting God's name . . . in that ordinary airplane terminal turned into a sacred sanctuary.

Lord, help me to always "see" with your eyes and be unhindered by my temporary trappings.

Reflections:

_____

_____

_____

_____

_____

JUNCTURE NINE

Who Is This?

"No one will be able to oppose you as long as you
live, for I will be with you just as I was with
Moses; I will not abandon you or fail to help you."
— (JOSH. 1:5, TLB)

Dementia insidiously crept into my world through my parents. First with my father, then my mother. Something revolutionary to my ability to cope with this unrelenting thief was to look at my parents through different lenses. When uncharacteristic and confusing actions and accusations took place, I had to remind myself of a simple truth. *It's the disease talking, not my dad. It's the disease talking, not my mom. It's the ugly disease talking; he never would have said that, she never would have said that. They never would have done that. It's the disease.*

For instance, when we first moved them to the assisted living facility. It was a nice place. Mom had a spacious bedroom, bathroom, living room/dining area. It was the disease talking when she called old friends and told them we had put her in one tiny little room, infested with rats. That wasn't her—*it was the disease talking.*

There was the time Dad had us duck down because we were being shot at by fighter planes flying by (in a hospital room). *That was the disease talking.*

Or when Mom would call one of my siblings to tell them things about me she didn't trust. *It was the disease.*

Or the day my father thought my mom was still married to her first husband, and he had just stopped by to drop off some books. He patted Mom's arm and said, "I can be your friend, but I can't be your husband" (it was devastating, and Mom was hysterical). They had been married for nearly fifty years. But we knew it was the Alzheimer's talking.

These occurrences can sometimes be humorous, sometimes sad, sometimes hurtful, uncomfortable, or even frightening. They can be nonsensical, or sound plausible, but not accurate. If you remind yourself often, "*it is the disease talking,*" it will make these situations more understandable and definitely more bearable to navigate.

Always remember: as our loved ones become harder to recognize, God, without fail, gives the courage and strength to maneuver through each situation.

Jesus, thank you for your never-ending presence and direction as we walk through this disease.

Reflections:

_____

_____

_____

_____

_____

JUNCTURE TEN

Always a Preacher

"Have I not commanded you? Be strong
and courageous. Do not be afraid; do not be
discouraged, for the Lord your God will be with
you wherever you go."
— (JOSH. 1:9, NIV)

Preacher, minister, pastor, or reverend, he carried those titles with revered awe. Once he accepted God's call, he never looked back. For my father, preaching was in his DNA— it was entwined in his every breath. Preacher was who he was, it was what defined him. The great ugliness of Alzheimer's is that it slowly strips away the trappings of life, one by one by one. With the passing of time, known, common functions, places, or events are lost. With my father, the last known items to go, that were as common as blinking, were praying and preaching.

It was a certified nursing assistant, or CNA, who spoke with me. She told me it would happen at mealtimes. My father would see all the folks gathered for the dinner. He didn't know where he was, but he saw people coming in and sitting down. For nearly fifty years, he had stood in the church and watched people coming in and sitting down. In his Alzheimer's afflicted brain, people coming in and sitting down equals CHURCH! In that locked unit, in the stuffy little cafeteria, when the other patients would gather for the meals, my father would stand up and he would preach! He would exhort during breakfast. He would expound at lunch, and he would dissect entire sermons while they were eating their dinner. He was so intent on delivering the message that the staff would bring him a little podium to preach from!

What is most amazing is that the young nurse sharing this with me told me how much she learned, and how it helped her. Wow! God was speaking through my father, through Alzheimer's, in the dining room, in the locked wing of the institution, and His voice was heard! God is with us in all circumstances, in all situations. He will never leave us alone.

Jesus, thank you and praise you for being so beautifully visible in the midst of these difficult days. You are my strength!

Reflections:

_____

_____

_____

_____

_____

Blissfully Unaware

"The fear of the Lord leads to life; then one rests
content, *untouched by trouble."*
— (PROV. 19:23, NIV)

After a time, the Alzheimer's sufferer becomes "blissfully unaware" of his/her surroundings. The trappings of this world and the present reality fade away. And although it is difficult on those observing, life becomes quite simple for the one carrying the disease.

Because my father was always restless and wandering, he was in a locked unit of the assisted-living facility. Long passed were the days of frustration, knowing he was having some memory trouble and aware things were not right. He was beginning to live in an "alternate reality," almost as though he had entered *The Twilight Zone.* He didn't know *where* he was, or *when* it was, or even some days *who* he was. Most of his days were now spent meandering through the halls of the facility, not being able to go beyond the locked and gated boundaries. Or sitting for long periods of time looking at nothingness. Or being corralled into the activity room or dining room for some interaction with other folks in the same condition.

On one particular day, we were visiting with him and trying to have a conversation. I asked, "So, Dad, what have you been doing today?" He clasped his hands behind his head and leaned back in his chair. Then with a contented sigh and happy smile, he replied, "I drove the truck to McDonald's and had a hamburger!"

We were glad he was content. Glad that he was blissfully unaware of his circumstances, limitations, and complete inability to leave the facility—much less drive a vehicle and get a hamburger! We were happy that he was happy. Oh, to be so sure and blissfully unaware! God brings such beautiful moments in the midst of heartache.

Thank you, Jesus, for giving us contentment in turmoil and simplicity in strife.

Reflections:

_____
_____
_____
_____

JUNCTURE TWELVE

Nice to See You

*"When you pass through the waters, I will be
with you; And through the rivers, they will not
overwhelm you. When you walk through fire, you
will not be scorched, nor will the flame burn you."*
— (ISA. 43:2, AMP)

"Meet them where they are." The facility Dad was in
had a motto to that effect. Meaning, join them
in their reality. Many moments, times, and days the person
with the disease is not aware of the current state of the
world. They are only aware of the world they are currently
in. It is infinitely better to join them than to try to coax or
argue them out of their present mindset.

My husband and I had gone to spend some time with
Dad in the locked unit of the Alzheimer's wing. We arrived
toward the end of a social gathering. Most of the residents

were in the activity room sitting around tables. The activity was finished, and they were eating cookies and had little cups of juice to drink. Dad had a pleasant look on his face and was very pleased to see us. We were just getting seated when the activity director announced it was over and everyone was free to go. The three of us were first to walk out. Then something very special happened. Dad stopped, turned around, and began shaking hands with the next person out of the door. Then the next, and the next, and the next. He was saying, "So good to see you today," "thank you for coming," "have a good week," and "God bless you." In that moment he wasn't diseased, he wasn't sick, and he wasn't locked in an institution for his safety. He was Rev. Lee McCleery, greeting the folks on their way out of church! Just like he had done thousands of times in his lifetime. He was in church and simply doing what he always did. My husband and I stood on either side of him and shook hands too! The people in that facility who were also locked in, each suffering from their own afflictions, walked out the door feeling as though they had just left church as well! They each had a smile on their face, having been warmly greeted by the pastor. It was beautiful.

Thank you, Jesus, for reminding us you are always there. And that you are the church triumphant, even in Alzheimer's disease.

Reflections:

_____

_____

_____

_____

_____

_____

JUNCTURE THIRTEEN

Is This My Balance?

". . . the wise bring calm . . ."
— (Prov. 29:11, NIV)

*"When I worried about many things, your assuring
words soothed my soul."*
— (Ps. 94:19, GW)

Well into the disease, my father had an appointment
with the neurologist. Before he was completely
confined, never to go out again, taking Dad out in public
became a very stressful situation for me. Not for him—for
him it was a delight! For me he was unpredictable, quick
on his feet, and didn't follow my directions. For him it was
a fun field trip! For me I had to keep one eye on him at
all times—while driving, parking, checking in, and praying
that he didn't need to use the restroom. For him it was a
grand adventure!

On this particular day we walked into the building, I assigned him a chair, and asked him to stay. I would be right there to sit with him. He asked me if they had his account balance. The reception area of the neurologist's office was set up in a bank-teller type of configuration. He thought we were at the bank. I told him I would check on it and be right back. As I was checking him in, he was suddenly beside me. He leaned past me and asked the young receptionist if she had his balance. Trying to help her understand, I explained that he was looking for his balance since we were at the bank. I assumed situations such as this must happen on occasion since we were at a neurologist's office. Her eyes widened— she looked at both of us in shock, amazement, and a little fear, pushed back in her chair and said absolutely nothing! I got the impression she thought we both had a problem! Her response surprised me and also elevated my stress level. I didn't know how long I could keep dad from getting his "balance." I told him we would get it in a minute and we sat down. I was nervously trying to keep him occupied while we waited our turn. Those minutes of waiting seemed like an eternity, and he really wanted to know his "balance."

His name was called, and we went into the exam room. The nurse was routinely asking the general questions, taking his weight, blood pressure, and writing it all down on her information sheet. As she was finishing up, Dad said, "Is that my balance?" She looked up, and it took her only a moment to understand, assess, and react. She said, "Yes, would you like it?" Dad nodded, and she handed it to him. He looked it all over (his weight, blood pressure, medications, etc.), and she asked if it looked okay. He said it was, contentedly folded it, and tucked it into his shirt pocket as I had seen him do countless times in my life. In that seemingly simple gesture, that nurse accomplished much. She treated my father with grace, respect, and dignity. She understood his illness. She completely dissipated my stress and gave me a calm assurance that I wasn't alone. She was the "balance" Dad and I both needed, and God put her in our path that day. She was the "wise that brought us calm."

Thank you, Jesus, for using others to show us your calm, and your assurance. And for the reminder that you can bring us "balance" in the unpredictable world of Alzheimer's disease. Let me hear your words that soothe my soul.

Reflections:

_____

_____

_____

_____

_____

JUNCTURE FOURTEEN

Traveling Companion

*"Don't be impatient for the Lord to act! Keep
traveling steadily along his pathway and in due
season he will honor you with every blessing."*
— (Ps. 37:34, NLT)

*"You see me when I **travel** and when I rest at
home. You know everything I do."*
— (Ps. 139:3, NLT)

Alzheimer's dementia is a progressive disorder. It steals the memory and functioning of its victims. Sometimes it seems to go rabbit fast, sometimes tortoise slowly. From one day to the next, a lifetime of cemented memories can be lost. It is a life-changing journey for everyone.

My two brothers had not seen our dad since he had been moved to the locked unit of the assisted-living facility.

Each brother lived in a different state far away, and both made the trip to be together when they saw Dad for the first time in this new phase of the journey. I tried to prepare them for the decline they would see in him. They chose to go together, just them, to see him for the first time. I waited expectantly in the hall on the other side of the imposing locked door.

When they emerged some time later, they were full of mixed emotions. Sadness and tears were first, then an amazed and somber realization of how difficult the situation had become. Lastly, they were tickled and squabbling over how the visit ended!

This is what they relayed to me. When they entered Dad's room, he was delighted to see them! He welcomed them, and hugged them, and wanted to talk to them all about their lives, jobs, and families. They discussed familiar topics with him that they knew would interest him, and he could talk about. It was a very pleasant visit. Each of my brothers has a great sense of humor and they use it liberally! It had been a successful encounter! As they were getting ready to leave, they asked Dad if he would pray for them. He readily assented. They stood, held hands, and Dad began his prayer. He boomed, "Lord, thank you for this day. Thank you for this wonderful visit, and I pray that you will give safe travels to my son and his travelling companion." They both looked at each other and said, "I'M THE SON!"

They were completely unaware until that moment that Dad didn't know BOTH of them were his sons. The joke and mystery in our family is still, "Which one was the son? And which one was the traveling companion?"

> *Thank you, Jesus, that we don't have to wonder who is our Traveling Companion! Thank you for the assurance that you are walking beside us each step of this journey, and we are confident that we are your sons and daughters.*

Reflections:

_____
_____
_____
_____
_____

JUNCTURE FIFTEEN

Nine Lives

*"Blessed be the God and Father of our Lord Jesus
Christ, the God of all comfort. He comforts us in
all our affliction, so that we may be able to comfort
those who are in any kind of affliction, through the
comfort we ourselves receive from God."*
— (2 Cor. 1:3–4, CSB)

Feelings are real. Alzheimer's is a memory disease. Whatever happens to affect the memory and rational thought are effects of the disease, resulting in continued diminished functioning in everyday life. But the feelings and emotions that come alongside are real and although will most likely dissipate shortly, they cannot be dismissed. They must be addressed. A lingering emotion is loneliness. So much has been lost, taken, or disappeared.

Some decisions have long-lasting ramifications. Mom was terribly lonely. Dad was vanishing before her eyes—she was separated by locked doors from him. Her living space had been reduced to three rooms (albeit comfortable, very nice rooms). She was confused, lost, and extremely lonely. I decided she needed a companion.

I got her a cat. A real cat. A live cat. A cat that needed food, water, a litter box, and care. It was a good idea in theory. She liked the idea. I thought it would keep her company. She agreed. I thought it would take minimal care. She thought she could care for it. I thought she would like it. She thought she would too. I was wrong on all accounts.

A trip to the humane society, and an admonition that we should get a full grown, litter-trained, mellow feline resulted in a scrawny, adorable, tiny, black kitten bearing the name of my brother, Marcus. She was in love.

Mom was incapable of the responsibility. She fed him cat treats instead of his food and couldn't clean up the inevitable messes. I arrived one day to the two of them sharing a lollipop. A lollipop! Mom took a lick; Marcus the Cat took a lick! Seriously?! She told me he loved it! That's when I knew this hadn't been the best idea, and I truly wondered if the cat would survive.

The answer came a mere five weeks after obtaining the little kitty. I was driving Mom to a doctor appointment and she said, "Joni, I don't want the cat anymore." I assured her it was fine, and I would take care of it. I just thought he would keep her company.

Marcus the Cat currently lives at my house. He has for several years now. And probably will for many more. He is a sweet cat and very easy to care for. He is a constant reminder of our Alzheimer days and how I wanted so desperately to sooth my mother's loneliness.

The cat was worth it. Completely worth it.

Jesus, we know that ultimate comfort and companionship comes from you. Thank you for giving us wisdom and ways to lend comfort. Help us remember to be understanding and patient with the emotions of our afflicted loved ones.

Reflections:

_____

_____

_____

_____

_____

JUNCTURE SIXTEEN

The Last Best Day

"Now thanks be to God for His indescribable gift
[which is precious beyond words]!"
— (2 COR.9:15, AMP)

When experiencing the decline of a loved one with dementia, some days you may be aware of a new symptom or forgotten occurrence, and some days it is so subtle and gradual that you look back and don't know when it happened. Then there may be a day in which something momentous occurs.

September 25, 1959, was my parents' wedding day. My mother had been a widow for a little over a year, with two young children. On that September afternoon long ago, my father chose to, "love, honor, and cherish" all three of them. I relish the pictures of that happy time. The beginning of a new family, new ministry, and great days ahead together. A few years later, after myself and my younger brother were born, our family picture was completed.

My parents spent nearly fifty years actively in ministry. Wherever God sent them, they sowed seeds of His love, mercy, forgiveness, and faithfulness. They were an inspiring and exemplary team.

September 25, 2009: my parents' fiftieth anniversary. My father was in a locked facility, slipping daily deeper into the Alzheimer's world of not knowing. We couldn't really take him out anymore because he could disappear so quickly, or have trouble in the restroom, or any number of problems we couldn't even foresee. But it was their fiftieth anniversary, and I wanted to honor my parents.

I decided to hold a little reception at the church. I thought if I could have it on a weekday, and invite the senior adults, there would be minimal chances of a disaster. If we could bring Dad over, keep him in one room for just a couple of hours, and take him right back, it might work!

On the prescribed day, we set our plan into motion. We had cake and punch and flowers. We had their wedding album. My mom was so excited. Folks from the church who hadn't met him showed up, and his sisters and brother came from out of state. Then Dad arrived. I was a nervous wreck. I didn't want anything to happen to diminish his dignity (always one of my biggest fears). I need not have worried.

God gave us a fabulous gift that day. Dad was inexplicably lucid and clear. His eyes were focused. He could communicate. He recognized his family. He smiled for all the pictures. He didn't seem terribly confused. In fact, he was so engaged that some people weren't sure that anything was wrong! It was miraculous! For those two hours we had a beautiful reprieve in the midst of the hardship. We know it was a marvelous, undeserved gift from our loving, heavenly Father to give us "the last best day" with our precious earthly father.

I will always cherish, "the last best day" I had with my dad.

Thank you, Jesus, for constantly ministering to us.
Thank you for the special gifts you give in the midst
of the valley. We cherish them.

Reflections:

_____
_____
_____
_____
_____

JUNCTURE SEVENTEEN

Stronger Than You Know

"Don't be afraid, for I am with you. Don't be discouraged, for I am your God. I will strengthen you and help you. I will hold you up with my victorious right hand."
— (Isa. 41:10, NLT)

As the dementia progresses, you will find it ever more necessary to be a frequent intercessor on behalf of your loved one. He/she may be completely unaware of your interceding, or may be resentful of your intrusion, as some other family members may feel. You, the caregiver, know what is happening, how it is progressing, what is possible and impossible. For a time you may not be the most popular person in your family, or in the facility, or wherever you are, but you must hold fast to the dedication of protecting the one afflicted with this debilitating disease. It is a hard and lonely place. But with God's sustaining grace, you are stronger than you know.

Always around Christmas. The festive season seemed to be when Mom would get exceptionally sick. It was just so hard. She very quickly had succumbed to pneumonia. It was late at night, and I made my way to the hospital to spend some (more) time with her.

As I was sitting, observing, praying, and wondering if she would recover this time, I noticed something unusual. She wasn't wearing her pain patch. Now she had been wearing pain patches for years at this point. Mom's pain stemmed from debilitating arthritis and osteoporosis. Daily, excruciating pain had been her companion for many, many years. The highly powerful, narcotic pain patches served to mostly relieve her of the hurt. Her body was used to the medication, it was dependent on it. The patch was missing. I was more than concerned—I was a bit panicky. Why was it not there? I found the nurse and asked why Mom was minus the pain patch. She informed me that the on-call doctor had instructed her to remove it—it was too high a dose of medication. Oh, no. Oh, no.

I was immediately overcome with a barrage of emotions. Fear, frustration, and the overwhelming sense of protection that I needed to give my mother. MY mother, the one who had birthed, raised, and protected ME. It was my turn. Although, I had been taught that doctors were the final authority on medical knowledge, and taught never to question their judgment, I knew I had to get that patch on my mother. If I didn't, she would be writhing in excruciating withdrawal pain—pain that I think would have been the end of her. I couldn't stomach the thought of witnessing such an event.

I was shaking, yet I insisted on calling the doctor myself. The nurse wasn't too happy. I think it was a breach of protocol. I didn't care. I had one all-consuming thought: "Keep Mom out of pain and alive." Thus, very late that December night I found myself on the phone with him, the doctor, who didn't know my mom, didn't know her history, didn't know her condition, and didn't understand why she was wearing such a powerful pain patch. I clearly and calmly gave him all of the reasons why she needed it. After some discussion, he obliged, he changed his order, and had the nurse re-apply it. I was still shaking, yet enormously relieved.

I was so thankful for the continuity of my precious mother's pain management, of her childlike trust in me, and of the strength only God can give a daughter to be the advocate Mom needed, that night, at that moment.

Jesus, please be our intercessor and advocate. Give us your strength, and work on our behalf when we are unaware of our circumstances. Thank you for your fortifying presence.

Reflections:

_____

_____

_____

_____

_____

There Is a Balm

*"Is there no **balm** in Gilead? Go up to Gilead to*
find balm for your wounds,"
— (JER. 8:22A, NIV; 46:10A)

"The fruit of [The Lord's] righteousness will be
***peace**; its effect will be quietness and confidence*
forever."
— (ISA. 32:17, NIV)

Alzheimer's disease can inflict insecurity, confusion, fearfulness, paranoia, and other unsettling and uncharacteristic emotions. The sufferer needs you, the caregiver, to be the calm, reassuring presence in their daily life of uncertainty.

Dignified, full of Integrity, brilliant, scholar, proud, humble, devoted husband and father, man of God. Just a few phrases and descriptive words I can attribute to my dad during his lifetime. They didn't quite apply to the Alzheimer's victim he became. Words for that version of my father were: unsure, lost, confused, frustrated, wanderer, sometimes violent, and unknowing. As he became increasingly more of the second description, some days became chaotic.

It was on many of these days, but one in particular, when my husband Doug had gone over to check on Dad. My precious father was wandering aimlessly through the locked corridors that now comprised his living space, and he was causing some consternation with other residents when Doug showed up. My loving husband corralled Dad back to his room and told him he was going to read some Scripture. Dad didn't really talk anymore, but he nodded and settled down a bit. Doug began to read. He read Joshua 1:8, "Keep this Book of the Law always on your lips; meditate on it day and night, so that you may be careful to do everything written in it. Then you will be prosperous and successful." Doug could sense the presence of the Lord. He knew Dad was listening. Verse 9: "Have I not commanded you? Be strong and courageous. Do not be afraid; do not be discouraged, for the Lord your God will be with you wherever you go." Dad was calming down. Doug moved on to Psalm 23, "The Lord is my shepherd . . . he leads me beside quiet waters, he refreshes my soul." Dad was visibly less tense, peaceful, and calm. Doug continued to read Psalm 28, "The Lord is my strength and my shield; my heart trusts in him, and he helps me."

Dad continued to relax. The calming, peaceful presence of God was palpable in that cramped, confined, and confusing nursing-home room.

When Doug thought maybe he had read enough, he stopped. Dad reached over and, looking clearly and lucidly into Doug's eyes, patted softly the beloved Book, and spoke the first words that had been spoken in many weeks: "Read more." Doug read more.

There is a Balm in Gilead . . . His name is Jesus.

> *Thank you, Jesus, that you are the Healing Balm*
> *that soothes our weary and frightened souls.*
> *Continue to remind us, you are the Balm in*
> *Gilead.*

Reflections:

_____

_____

_____

_____

_____

JUNCTURE NINETEEN

A New Song

*"But I will **sing** of your strength, in the morning I*
*will **sing** of your love; for you are my fortress, my*
refuge in times of trouble."
— (Ps. 59:16, NIV)

"Sing *to the Lord a new song; **sing** to the Lord, all*
*the earth. **Sing** to the Lord, praise his name."*
— (Ps. 96:1–2, NIV)

Music is seemingly one of the last strongholds of memories our bodies give up, with much resistance. From our earliest days, music in some way has impacted our lives, and it is stored into deep, armored vaults in our minds. An Alzheimer's sufferer can sometimes be reached, soothed, or rallied a bit with the power of a melody.

Our church had a small ensemble from the choir that would visit the "hospice house" weekly in town. They sang hymns and songs of hope for the patients and their families to comfort them in their last and difficult days. One warm July evening, the group chose to go to my dad's place and sing expressly for him. They brought in the keyboard, set it up, and squeezed eight folks into the room. Dad slumped in the recliner, head down, mute, with eyes clouded, as they began to sing. When the familiar tunes saturated his senses, the transformation was incredible. He sat up, lifted his head, eyes focused on the group, smiled, and began to sing along to the old hymns and songs he had known for decades. He was praising and glorifying his Savior! It was amazing. What happened next was even more astonishing. The leader asked Dad if he had any requests. I thought, "That's ridiculous. He doesn't know what's going on. There's no way he could give a request. Plus, he's not talking." About the time I was done thinking that, Dad said, "Do you have any Christmas songs?" I was in awe. The leader said, "Sure, we can sing Christmas songs in July!" And so we did! Dad sang along with each familiar carol, and every one of us had a holy moment with our Savior—the One who causes us to sing. That evening I gained a fresh perspective on the psalmist's words, "Sing to the Lord a <u>new</u> song."

In that encounter, I believe I was privileged to glimpse a bit of the heavenly host singing,

*"Glory to God in the highest
and on earth peace to those on whom his favor rests."*

*Jesus, help me to always "sing a new song" to you.
Thank you that you are my fortress and my refuge
in times of trouble. I sing praises to your name.*

Reflections:

_____

_____

_____

_____

_____

JUNCTURE TWENTY

Gratitude

*"I was thirsty, and you gave me something to drink
. . . I tell you, whatever you did for one of the least
of these, you did for me."*
— (MATT. 25:35, 40, NIV)

One of the great difficulties of caregiving for the one consumed by Alzheimer's is ascertaining certain physical problems. As communication ability is diminished, common ailments can become more pronounced and severe. It is much like trying to decipher what is wrong with a small child who is unable to understand or verbalize what is happening to them.

Dad was in the hospital. A portion of his Alzheimer's journey took him to a specialized facility in a small town on the Kansas prairie. Then he became ill and was admitted to the county hospital. It was a forty-five-minute drive from my house. Every day that he was there, I drove out and sat by him. It was really hard. In addition to the numerous ways I was losing my father through this awful disease, to see him physically sick was tough. I sat with him to be his eyes, his ears, his barometer of feeling. I was his voice for the nurses and doctor. I was his advocate. When I was overwhelmed with the heartache and responsibility, I would go to the end of the hall in a little waiting room to cry and pray. God would buoy me, wrap me in His love, strengthen me, and I would go back to sit with Dad.

One moment, one time, one day, Dad indicated he was thirsty. It was the only understood communication I had had from him for a while. I immediately jumped up, got the cup of water and handed it to him. He guzzled it through the straw as though he hadn't had a drink in days! When he was finished, he gave a satisfied "Ahhh." Then he turned, looked up at me and said, "Thank you." For the span of time it took to say those two simple words of gratitude, there was a transformation. I was the daughter giving my dad a drink, so commonplace, so mundane, so "normal"— yet so utterly miraculous!

In that moment God showered me with the refreshing, rejuvenating, life-giving water that only He can give. In that briefest moment of gratitude from my earthly father, I was overwhelmed with the presence of my heavenly Father! I will always be grateful for that restorative moment.

Gracious, heavenly Father, with an overflowing heart of gratitude, I thank you for your life-giving water and your presence, which gives me the strength to face another day. Thank you.

Reflections:

_____

_____

_____

_____

_____

JUNCTURE TWENTY-ONE

Repeat-Repeat-Repeat

*"For the Lord gives skillful and godly wisdom; from
His mouth come knowledge and understanding."*
— (PROV. 2:6 AMP)

A relatively common attribute or symptom of dementia is repetition. The person with the disease will repeat, repeat, repeat the same sentence, story, phrase, or question. If you, the caregiver, do not understand this ramification of the disease, it can become a frustrating occurrence for both you and your loved one. A simple, yet effective way to help alleviate or diffuse the frustration of the situation is to divert or redirect the conversation or change the focus of their attention.

Mom repeated herself a lot. She would say something, then turn away, and in a moment, turn back, and say the exact same thing over again, in the same words, and the same tone. She would leave several identical messages in the voicemail on our phones. I once counted seventeen times that she told my daughter McKenna she liked her new haircut. I wondered how many times she would say it without some type of intervention, so I just counted. Seventeen. "McKenna, your hair looks nice." "Thanks, Gram, I just got it cut." Seventeen times. My dear girl was so patient and sweet. For all seventeen.

We were in a lobby, waiting for a pulmonologist, Dr. Wong. We spent much time in doctors' waiting areas. Mom was in a wheelchair, subdued, and watching the floor. She happened to look up and see Dr. Wong's name on the wall. She read his name out loud, more loudly than I would have liked, "Dr. Wong." Then turning to me, in a voice definitely more loudly than I would have liked, she said, "Do you think he is Oriental?" I was mortified! "Yes, Mother, I believe he is Asian," I said while trying to make the point about how socially incorrect her statement was in the middle of the lobby with people all around us. She responded, "Oh," and slumped back down. I tried to slump down, too, and be invisible.

About two minutes later, she looked up, saw his name on the wall and once again, read it out loud—and again, too loud: "Dr. Wong, do you think he is Oriental?" Oh, my goodness! I was mortified for the second time! I again replied as I did before, "Yes Mother, he is Asian." And once again, she responded, "Oh," and slumped back down in the wheelchair.

I knew then that if I didn't redirect her, or the conversation, we were in a cycle. And definitely a cycle I didn't want to be in! I jumped up and turned her wheelchair one-hundred-and-eighty degrees so that her back was at the wall. Situation solved! Whew! All of the stress, frustration, and embarrassment was quickly and efficiently diffused for me, and Mom was perfectly protected.

Jesus, thank you for the insight to know how to care
for my loved one in new and uncharted situations.
You give wisdom and grace that overwhelms me.

Reflections:

_____
_____
_____
_____
_____

JUNCTURE TWENTY-TWO

Clear!

*"All the words of my mouth are right and good.
There is nothing in them that is against the
truth. They are all clear to him who understands,
and right to those who find much learning. Take
my teaching instead of silver. Take much learning
instead of fine gold."*
— (Prov. 8:8–10, NIV)

There are several types of dementia. My father was diagnosed with two, which is not uncommon. The first being Alzheimer's, and the second Lewy body. For an abbreviated definition of Lewy body dementia, it can be characterized as the one in which the sufferer hallucinates. The hallucinations can range from mild and sometimes humorous, to dark and terrifying. The unseen objects/events my dad experienced fell into every category in the range, from seeing a kangaroo hop across the room, to war and death.

During my teenage years, my dear father was able to fulfill one of his greatest dreams in life. He learned to fly. It was a lofty and extravagant wish that he never thought he could afford to achieve as a pastor. But God gave him an opportunity. He didn't go to flight school, he just read the manual and took the test and passed! Smart guy! We had a church member who owned a single-engine, four-seater, Cessna 172 and offered it free for Dad's actual flight training. It's a period of time in my life when I can remember seeing my dad really happy about something. He was nearly ecstatic, giddy with the ability to defy gravity and soar with the eagles!

When a pilot of a small plane is getting ready for takeoff, there is a checklist that is meticulously followed, with the final step being a call of, "Clear!" out of the window, just prior to taxiing down the runway. I can still hear/see him, all smiles as he opened that window and yelled, "Clear!" And away we went!

Thirty years later I was walking in a small, closed-in, gated (locked), courtyard with Dad. It was a warm, late spring day, and we were circling the bushes on the never-ending ovular pathway. Dad looked up into the bright, cloudless blue sky and said, "Look at the plane." I looked and saw nothing, so (to make sure of myself), I asked him where it was, and he pointed directly overhead at nothing but bright blue sky and said, "Right there." In my love and respect for him, (plus the bit of knowledge that it's better to meet him in his reality), I said, "Oh, yes, there it is." Then for the next few minutes our little closed-in, gated, monotonous path became an airport—and a runway! His lethargy fell away, his countenance brightened, and he came alive! He walked me through each step of the approach, the banking, turning, the lowering of the flaps, landing gear, and we guided that nonexistent plane to land right at our feet, complete with Dad having me step back out of the way! For those brief, bright moments, the word "Clear!" took on a whole new meaning. In his disease-ridden mind and body, he was "clear," and God gave us a sacred moment in that tiny courtyard.

Lord, help me see clearly and understand your working during this season. Thank you for always being, "Clear!"

Reflections:

_____

_____

_____

_____

_____

JUNCTURE TWENTY-THREE

The Essence of a Life

"But it is the spirit in a person, the breath of the
*Almighty, that gives them **understanding**."*
— (JOB 32:8, NIV)

Alzheimer's steals a person's memories, steals their ability to function as they once did. It steals great quantities of life's day-to-day living. But it doesn't always steal the essence of a person. It's still in there—not always visible, but occasionally surfacing. Those are treasured moments, gifts from God.

For a vocation and lifetime my father was a pastor. But he was much more than that at home. Dad was a carpenter. He was a fix-it guy. He worked his way through college by building houses. He appreciated fine craftsmanship. As a child I never remember a plumber, electrician, or handyman ever stepping foot into our house. Dad could remedy any problem. He had an entire arsenal of tools and gadgets to correct or build whatever was needed or wanted. His favorite tool of all time was a giant lathe, not only wood-turning, but metal-turning. He made hundreds of items and gifts from that hulking machine. He delighted in the precision of the cuts and grooves he turned using the lathe. He was so proud of his ability, and he was very particular. He wanted each creation to be as close to perfect as possible.

We walked daily through the assisted-living facility trying to process what was happening with my father and trying to console and comfort my mother with her confusion and anxiety. He was unable to speak coherently—he just walked, and walked, and walked. He was in the locked wing for his safety. As we aimlessly roamed the hallways, I began to notice something interesting that Dad did regularly. When we passed by a table, or a bench, or a chair, he would reach out and run his hand over the wood, just as I had seen him do hundreds of times when working with a piece or inspecting some furniture to examine its quality. Sometimes he would stop, wordlessly admiring the grain and assessing the precision of the corners and legs. He would even occasionally get on the floor and look underneath to see if it had been constructed to his standards! Although he was unable to communicate verbally, it was clearly evident when his years of woodworking, building, and fixing would overtake him. We could see and sense the essence of him—it was still there, deep inside, and we cherished those moments. They were special.

Lord, give me understanding, help me see the
essence of my loved one . . .

Reflections:

_____
_____
_____
_____
_____

JUNCTURE TWENTY-FOUR

Divine Dementia

*"His divine power has given us everything we need
for a godly life through our knowledge of him who
called us by his own glory and goodness."*
— (2 PETER 1:3, NIV)

Professional. Dignified. Stately. That was Dad. He was
serious about his obligation to God. He was always the
best version of himself in public. He wore a suit and tie
to the office every day. When he stood behind the pulpit
on Sunday morning as God's vessel, his suit was black,
always black, with an understated tie. Every Sunday. He was
groomed meticulously. He never wanted his appearance to
hinder the message he was charged with. It was his passion.
It was his purpose. He was humbled and awed that God had
called *him*. He would represent God with his best, down
to his freshly shined wing-tipped shoes. I surmise there are

many, many people during the course of his ministry who never saw him in relaxation mode, wearing jeans, shorts, or tennis shoes.

As Alzheimer's was stealing him away, the ability to continue his dignified demeanor was lessening. Sometimes it seemed rapid, other times more gradual.

Dad's days in the final two years of his life were filled with endless shuffling, shuffling, shuffling, up and down hallways, in and out of others' rooms (much to their consternation). Wearing baggy sweatpants, an undershirt, and socks with no shoes, he spent his days locked in a facility, roaming aimlessly and endlessly. It was truly heartbreaking to witness.

On one particular day, as I was lamenting the evils of this nasty disease, I paused to take a breath, and God lovingly and ever so gently gave me a beautiful truth.

God revealed to me that Dad didn't know what was happening to him. He had no idea whatsoever the manner in which he spent his days, how he was unkempt and clothed perpetually in pajamas. He didn't know Alzheimer's was doing its best to strip him of his dignity. Dad didn't know what he had become. HE was not aware. WE were aware. WE were definitely, and painfully, aware. But HE was not. God had placed him in a cocoon of unknowingness.

I was, and am still to this moment, so incredibly, overwhelmingly grateful to my Friend, Jesus, for sparing my father the pain of the reality. As difficult as it was for us, Dad was not suffering with the knowledge of what was happening.

I like to think of it as his, "Divine dementia."

Thank you, Jesus, for your beautiful truth and protection, which gives us the ability to step into a new day.

Reflections:

_____

_____

_____

_____

_____

JUNCTURE TWENTY-FIVE

Honored

"And the peace of God [that peace which reassures the heart, that peace] which transcends all understanding, [that peace which] stands guard over your hearts and your minds in Christ Jesus [is yours]."
— (PHIL. 4:7, AMP)

"Honor your father and your mother, *so that you may live long in the land the Lord **your** God is giving you."*
— (EX. 20:12, NIV)

If you haven't discovered yet—you probably will soon—that being the caregiver comes with enormous pressures and responsibilities. It can also bring along relationship-altering choices. Especially with other family members (at least in my case).

At first, I listened politely to my siblings and relatives as they shared with me what I should/could/needed to be doing to provide the type of care my parents deserved. At first, I truly tried to implement their suggestions and acknowledge their concerns. At first, I really tried to keep everyone happy. As time went on and Dad, then Mom, became increasingly impaired, it was absolutely impossible to keep all the plates spinning. I had to make a choice.

I knew my choice would not be popular with everyone. But it was necessary. I believed God had placed the care of my parents in my hands. With His help I was determined to put their needs, their care, their well-being, and their protection above the uninformed or surmised thoughts of others who were hundreds of miles away. In those months and years, I was as protective as a mama bear. Only I knew what each day held. Only I witnessed the decline daily. Only I could make the most informed decisions. It was hard. It was scary. It was sad. It led to fractured family relationships.

Now my parents are both gone. I wish I could say things are better. Unfortunately, that is not the reality. Unfortunately, we have become a fractured family.

It was one of the greatest privileges of my life to honor my parents and the hardest thing I've ever done. And I would do it again. Without a moment's hesitation.

*Jesus, thank you for the peace you give in the
turmoil of life's most difficult circumstances. I pray
for your healing of our fractured family and broken
relationships. I ask for reconciliation.
I trust in you.*

Reflections:

_____
_____
_____
_____
_____

JUNCTURE TWENTY-SIX

Wings of Safety

*"You will be secure, because there is hope; you will look about you and take your rest in **safety**."*
— (JOB 11:18, NIV)

*"Let me live forever in your sanctuary, **safe** beneath the shelter of your wings."*
— (Ps. 61:4, NLT)

When the one with Alzheimer's has lost the ability to communicate, it becomes an enormous task for the caregiver to anticipate and decipher their needs. It is a task of constant study, observation, and understanding to identify the signs of want, need, or distress.

Her name was Deb. She was the first caregiver we met in the final nursing-home facility where Dad was placed. She was loud and brash. She was invasive of personal space. But she was confident of her ability to care for Dad.

We were visiting in the common room. Six of us and Deb. Dad was wandering around the room, unaware of our presence. We were engaged in conversation—I saw Dad walking beside the counter along the wall. Nothing unusual, nothing more. I was involved in the conversation at hand. Suddenly Deb jumped up, flew across the room, and got behind Dad just as his legs gave way and he fell right into her waiting arms, gentle as beautiful wings. It happened seemingly instantaneously. Deb said she had been watching and could tell his legs were wobbling, and she sensed he was about to fall. The rest of us had absolutely no idea— we would have watched him collapse before we were aware there was a problem.

Deb was an incredible, attentive, and beloved caregiver whom we trusted implicitly with my father and mother. She became another pair of eyes, hands, feet, and wings of love and safety for us during those difficult days.

Dear Jesus, please send those who can be the wings of safety for us, to help us during this tiresome journey. Thank you for the promise of hope, safety, and rest.

Reflections:

_____

_____

_____

_____

_____

JUNCTURE TWENTY-SEVEN

Tornado Alley

*"Then they cried out to the Lord in their trouble,
and he brought them out of their distress. He stilled
the storm to a whisper."*
— (Ps. 107:28–29, NIV)

There are "side effects" for us, the caregivers, to having a loved one in a nursing home. "Side effects" such as getting to know the other residents, especially those who have no visitors. "Side effects" such as getting to know the staff in every department: kitchen, activity director, nursing, administrative, social worker, occupational therapy, physical therapy, laundry, and transportation. A natural outcome of the "side effects" is ministry, touching lives, showing Jesus.

We lived in "Tornado Alley." Probably having a loved one in a nursing home in the middle of Kansas isn't the most ideal location. There are vicious storms and regular tornado threats. Nonetheless that is precisely where we were.

A storm was brewing. I was at the facility visiting a bit, as I was most days. On that particular day, my husband and three teenage children were with me. The skies were ominous, greenish gray and very still. A nurse reported a tornado watch in effect and closed the curtains to help maintain calm. Mom was getting nervous. (She had survived a savage, deadly tornado as a young wife and mother, tornadoes were especially terrifying for her). We tried keeping her distracted. A few minutes later, the nurse returned, stating it was a *tornado warning* (meaning one has been sighted, and is a real possibility of hitting our location). We had to move to the most secure location in the building, the cafeteria.

Moving a hundred or so elderly and infirmed folks during a potential tornado is a monumental engineering feat! Most are in wheelchairs, the remaining are using some type of walking device, and the others are confused, needing directions. All are anxious and can sense the stress of the handful of workers, trying to accomplish this monstrous task. They first moved all residents outside of their rooms to the hallways, it was a giant wheelchair traffic jam! Then, they began one by one, pushing them into the cafeteria. At that time, my little family sprang into action! All five of us were pushing folks into to the "safe room", to avoid the tornado. I was blessed to watch my teenage children willingly and confidently escort lonely, elderly, and frightened residents to safety. I listened as they chatted and calmed those precious folks.

Eventually, the entire facility relocated to the cafeteria. The storm was raging, the residents were still very anxious, nervous and fearful. The staff was distributing snacks and juice, trying to promote calm. It was a slight distraction, they were on edge and stressed too. There was palpable tension in the room.

What happened next was marvelous and magnificent! We had church! My husband began to lead some singing. He asked the residents what they wanted, "Amazing Grace", "How Great Thou Art", and "Great is thy Faithfulness" is what they wanted. During that storm, during that tornado warning, the tension eased, the Glorious Presence of God entered in, it fortified us, it calmed us, reassured us, and we had a praise meeting! The last song that day was, "Jesus Loves Me", sung with fearless passion, by resident, visitor, and staff alike! We had Church!

By then the storm had subsided, and all were safe. All were secure. All had been in the presence of Jehovah. Oh, the treasured, "side effects" of the journey.

Jesus, thank you for holding us in the storm. Thank you for the "side effects" of opportunities to show your love to others, while caring for our own.

Reflections:

_____

_____

_____

_____

_____

JUNCTURE TWENTY-EIGHT

Always New

*"The Lord's . . . tender compassions fail not. They
are new every morning; great and abundant is your
stability and faithfulness."*
— (Lam. 3:22–23, AMP)

One of the interesting qualities of Alzheimer's is its ability to bring the bearer into a simpler existence. It pares down the encumbrances of daily living and magnifies moments of beauty. But we, the caregivers, must choose to look for those moments.

Christmas in the nursing home. What do you give someone who doesn't even know it's Christmas? Why celebrate? What's the point? Why? Because ONE of history's two greatest events EVER occurred! Because your loved one has celebrated for decades. Because it will give a few moments of pleasure. Because you, the caregiver, need these moments.

My son found the little box in a thrift store. One dollar and ninety-nine cents. It was gold with a very unassuming red ribbon on top. But that little box was concealing a wonderful surprise! When the lid was removed, two sides of the box fell open, and a darling little nativity scene was revealed! It was a typical scene, Mary, Joseph, and baby Jesus were the prominent figures with the usual wise men, shepherds, and animals facing the manger. The figures were made of a kind of hardened clay, and they had a childlike countenance. We thought it would be an enjoyable addition to the few items we had gathered for Mom.

She had opened a couple of other gifts, then turned to the little gold box. When she lifted the lid and the sides fell down revealing the beautiful, familiar scene, she gasped and clutched her hands together in elation. There He was, Emmanuel, God with us. With tears in her eyes she exclaimed, "Oh, it's *my* Jesus! It's *my* Jesus!" She was overwhelmed!

One of the kids showed her how to close the box by putting the lid back on, and she set it to the side to open another gift. After a few moments, she looked over and spotted the little gold box. Having no recollection of it, Mom asked if she could open it! Why of course! When she lifted the lid and the sides fell down revealing the beautiful, familiar scene, she gasped and clutched her hands together in elation, just as she did before. There He was Emmanuel, God with us. With tears in her eyes she exclaimed a second time, "Oh, it's *my* Jesus, It's *my* Jesus!" Once again, she was overwhelmed!

As before, the children assisted their dear Grandma in putting on the lid of the box and setting it to the side. A few moments later, she saw the little gold box again . . .

This perfect rhythm of worship, joy, and adoration for our Savior, Emmanuel, was repeated several more times, with Mom reacting identically every time! Seeing HER Jesus was wonderful, exhilarating, rapturous—and always new.

Oh, Emmanuel, give me a childlike spirit to see
you every day as though it were my first glimpse of
your glory. I praise and thank you for being "always
new." You are my Jesus! My Jesus!

Reflections:

_____
_____
_____
_____
_____

JUNCTURE TWENTY-NINE

Winter Fruit

"Then the angel showed me the river of the water of life. The river was shining like crystal. It flows from the throne of God and of the Lamb down the middle of the street of the city. The tree of life was on each side of the river. It produces fruit twelve times a year, once each month. The leaves of the tree are for the healing of all people."
— (REV. 22:1–2, ICB)

When a loved one is suffering from dementia, there can be several clues to determine whether it is dementia or simply normal aging. One such clue is through the sense of sight. When the brain is sending inaccurate information to the eyes, the individual must make a "best guess" at what they are seeing. This causes difficulty in identifying objects and people. It also causes the inability to keep track of dates, seasons, and the passage of time. Time becomes inconsequential.

The absence of time. Sounds like the beginning of eternity to me.

The Winter King Hawthorn is known as a four-season tree. In spring this hardy tree shows off pretty white flowers, lush dark leaves in summer, turning beautiful golden yellow in fall. The little berries it produces start out green, then orange, and by late fall and winter, are a luxurious red. Birds and small mammals are grateful for the sustenance these little berries provide throughout the cold months. The older branches are silvery gray and shimmer majestically in the winter sunlight. The Winter King will grow in poor soil, partial sun, heat, drought, and other inhospitable environments. It is a truly lovely tree.

Right outside Mom's window. That's where it was. That beautiful tree. She had the perfect view for the last few months on this earth—its graceful branches so close and ever-changing. That Winter King lived up to its name. I believe it was her prelude to eternity. In that unassuming, tenacious tree, growing in the lifeless Kansas dirt, she was drawing ever nearer to the King of Kings and the Tree of Life flourishing beside the Crystal River, bearing a new fruit each month.

Oh, did I tell you? She especially loved the "cherries" that grew in January. That may be her favorite "fruit of the month" in Glory Land.

Jesus, thank you for a glimpse and a reminder that
during our hardest days here, we have eternity,
where indescribable sights and experiences
await us.

Reflections:

_____
_____
_____
_____
_____

JUNCTURE THIRTY

Is it Contagious?

"Do not neglect your friend or your parent's friend
for that matter. When hard times come, you
don't have to travel far to get help from family; A
neighbor who is near is better than a brother who
is far away."
— (Prov. 27:10, Voice)

An "interesting" characteristic of dementia is how it affects each afflicted person differently. I'm not a scientist or an expert, but I have read some, and I have spent countless hours in the company of folks with varying forms and stages of dementia. Some become loud and flamboyant, some become shy and docile, others become violent and difficult, and some cry—a lot.

Her name was Katie. She was around my mother's age. Katie moved in across the hall from Mom during the last few months of my mother's life. She was a lovely Christian lady although, unfortunately, also suffering from Alzheimer's disease. Katie's daughter, much like myself, spent many hours with her mom at the nursing home. We became friends, Katie's daughter and I, bound by the commonality of what each of us was facing. We stood in the hallway and discussed at length the difficulties we each had while navigating the disease of our moms.

While Katie's daughter and I became friends, Katie and Mom became friends. It was an interesting and, at times, amusing friendship. My mom, keeping Katie company, would visit with her and "help" Katie make phone calls to her daughter (which ended up being the same call, repeated multiple times). Although Katie was very sweet, she was very sad and teary much of the time. It was a manifestation of her Alzheimer's. She was confused and upset at her surroundings, and it made her cry often. Actually, she cried a lot. My mom would do her best to comfort and console her. But with Mother's limited grasp of the situation, it would often frustrate her. One day as I was visiting, Mom was talking to me about Katie's ongoing sadness and her frustration as to why Katie would cry so often. I said, "You know, Mom, she has Alzheimer's" (thinking it might help her understand—silly me). She looked at me with consternation and quickly replied, "Oh, please pray I never get that!" I assured her I would. She didn't have the slightest inclination that it was too late, and we were way down the road on her own Alzheimer's journey. It was a beautiful reminder of how she was unaware of her situation and could be in a position to "help" her neighbor.

Thank you, Lord, for using Alzheimer's to bring unexpected friendships. Again, I am reminded of your presence always with us, through each experience and every day.

Reflections:

_____

_____

_____

_____

_____

JUNCTURE THIRTY-ONE

Hidden Treasure

*"I will give you hidden **treasures**, riches stored in
secret places, so that you may know that I am the
Lord, the God of Israel, who summons
you by name."*
— (ISA. 45:3 NIV)

While navigating Alzheimer's with your loved one,
you may discover something remarkable. Your loved
one may not know the day, month, year, what they ate for
breakfast, or even who you are, but it's possible they will
remember a skill or concept learned at a very young age.
And sometimes it just shows up.

Mom was the epitome of a model pastor's wife. I
believe if you ask those who knew her in that role, they
would agree. She was committed to doing anything to
enhance my father's ministry and further the kingdom of
Christ. She did it all. She was loving, friendly, and kind. She

wrote encouraging letters and made phone calls. She was a consummate teacher. She could teach teenagers, adults, or children. But children were her specialty! Mom could keep a room of a couple hundred children enthralled in rapt attention—she was incredible! There was no one to equal her. To see her in her prime was absolutely mesmerizing and awe inspiring. She could cook scrumptious meals and set the table as though she were entertaining royalty. It was always a privilege to be invited over to the McCleerys' house for Sunday dinner, because everyone knew it would be an unforgettable experience! And it was!

Also, along with all her other helpful pastor's wife attributes, she could play the piano! When she was a young pastor's wife, this gift was needed more often than in her later years. Subsequently, as she got older, folks didn't know this was a skill she possessed. I always loved hearing her play—it was strong, powerful, and energetic, just like her! My siblings and I called it, "saloon style."

Decades later on a sad, dreary day, we were in a facility visiting my father (he was moved a couple of times, always to a locked unit, and he was always heavily medicated). The weight of it was oppressive on all of us. Mom, crippled with arthritis, osteoporosis, and Alzheimer's, was slouched over, moving slowly down the corridor. My husband and children were also there with us. There was a piano sitting idle, and as we walked past, I asked Mom if she thought she could play something. I don't know why, but I asked her. She didn't know if she could, but she sat down on the bench. My children had no idea their precious Gram could play a single note.

A hymnal was on the rack, we opened it to, "How Great Thou Art," and she started playing, scarcely looking at the notes. It was a bit difficult with her arthritic fingers, but it was a glorious moment! My children were captivated. And amazed. We listened and sang along. We were all transported for a few minutes as the years and sickness melted away, and we were able to experience that "hidden treasure" and create a memory "to treasure" during the long days of Alzheimer's.

"Then sings my soul, my Savior God, to Thee . . ."

Jesus, thank you for bringing hidden treasures to the surface, for giving us moments we can enjoy in the midst of this difficult time. Thank you for once again reminding us, through a song played in a locked unit of a nursing home, through bent fingers, that you are here. How Great You Are.

Reflections:

_____

_____

_____

_____

Going Out

> *"You have let me experience the joys of life and the exquisite pleasures of your own eternal presence."*
> — (Ps. 16:11, TLB)

One of the beauties of Alzheimer's disease is the opportunity to experience "normal" life events without ever leaving the place where your loved one resides. It is fairly simple to change scenery—a walk down the hall, or in a courtyard—and feel as though you are in an altogether different place and enjoy some pleasant time together.

It was a nondescript conference room. There was a big ovular table with maybe eight chairs around it. This functional utilitarian set of four walls and a small window was no more than fifty feet from Mom's room in the nursing home. Just go left out her door, walk down the hall past the nurse's station, and there it was. To the right. It was empty most of the time.

We asked once if we could bring in some dinner for Mom and eat it in the conference room. Sure thing. Then we asked again. No problem. And again. Absolutely. And again. Of course. And again.

Something transformational happened each time we had dinner in the conference room. Whatever we brought in—subs, chicken, or burgers—the conference room became that restaurant. As soon as the door closed, we were "out" to the sub shop, or the chicken place, or the hamburger joint. Taking those few steps down the hall, bringing in something different, gave us a personal, relaxed, family-dinner time.

During the holidays the conference room became "home." I would set the table with linens and familiar dishes. We had Thanksgiving dinner, or our traditional Christmas chili, and New Year's Day lunch. These times were cherished moments for us. My family shared some precious, unforgettable, and happy times with Mom.

When the meal was done, when Mom was becoming tired, and it was time to go, we packed up and wheeled her back to her room. She had thoroughly enjoyed her time of "going out." As did we.

*Jesus, thank you for helping us find the bright
moments in the midst of this disease. Thank you for
the opportunity to "go out."*

Reflections:

_____
_____
_____
_____
_____

JUNCTURE THIRTY-THREE

Alzheimer's Blessing

"But as for me, it is good to be near God. I have
made the Lord God my safe place. So, I may tell of
all the things you have done."
— (Ps. 73:28, NLV)

Alzheimer's is a terrible disease. It is insipid. It is no respecter of person, race, religion, class, status, possessions, or anything. It preys on anyone. It can begin in nearly any decade of your life. It has been called "the long goodbye." It can stretch out for years in a person's life. It is difficult to diagnose at the beginning. It becomes clearer as it progresses. It is not a normal part of aging. It is an ugly, debilitating disease.

As I was living day to day with the reality of my father and mother's decline into the abyss of Alzheimer's, I had many conversations with God about it. He gently, lovingly, and gracefully gave me His comfort, along with some insights for which I am very grateful.

From what I witnessed, there seems to be little to nonexistent physical pain in Alzheimer's. It is not a painful disease. It does not fill one's body with pain. It doesn't target areas with pain. It is a disease of the brain, which greatly affects areas of the body (considering the brain is the control center), but not with physical pain.

I thank God for this revelation He gave me. I call it the blessing of Alzheimer's.

My mother lived for years with debilitating, excruciating arthritis and osteoporosis. Her fingers were gnarled, bones had collapsed in her back, and she was permanently stooped. Every day she fought to keep moving—it was a monumental battle. My first sentence to her for years was, "How is your pain today?" She would offer me a rundown of each area affected. Or I would ask what number from one to ten was she on the pain scale, and she would invariably reply, "eleven." (Kind of negated the pain scale thing.) She relied on massive doses of narcotic pain killers administered in the form of patches that needed to be replaced every three days, but regularly gave only minimal relief. I'd seen her thus heavily medicated, curled in a fetal position crying, still in unbearable agony.

As she was progressing further into Alzheimer's, there was a dramatic change. Monumental. Unbelievable.

Miraculous! When I asked her the question, "How is your pain today?" she would stop, cock her head to the side, think for a moment, and reply cheerfully, "It's good!" NO pain. NONE. She couldn't feel the arthritis in her hands, wrists, shoulders, hips, knees, and feet. No reminder of the broken bones and compressed vertebrae constantly screaming from her back. Alzheimer's removed her pain. Alzheimer's, this terrible, awful, damaging disease, released her from the physical agony she had endured for years.

How good and gracious is our God. I unashamedly declare this an Alzheimer's blessing!

Thank you, Jesus, for your gracious blessings
in the dark days.

Reflections:

_____

_____

_____

_____

_____

JUNCTURE THIRTY-FOUR

Holding On

"For I am the Lord your God who takes hold of
*your **right hand** and says to you, do not fear; I*
will help you."
— (Isa. 41:13 NIV)

One of the advantages of dementia is the ability to distract and redirect the afflicted. To redirect can generally diffuse a sticky situation. A change in the direction of a conversation or a new environment can lead to an unexpected, pleasant moment.

Redirecting may be fairly easily accomplished by taking our loved one "out." "Out" of their despondency, and "out" of their surroundings.

We discovered an ingenious way to take Mom "out" for the evening. Pizza and a movie. As my mother's world shrank to the confines of one room, a hospital bed, a few of her belongings, and a wheelchair, she couldn't venture very far. She would only leave her room when the staff came and wheeled her down for a meal, or sometimes an activity or fellowship, but generally she wasn't interested or able. Until we discovered "pizza and a movie." We learned that she would enjoy—and could kind of follow the storyline—of an animated children's film. We would order a pizza, pick it up, hot, fresh and greasy. We would choose a movie. And we would choose one our three teenage children. (It was never difficult for them. Each one was delighted to be with their Gram.) We would journey to the nursing home and, along with the pizza, drop off the chosen movie buddy. When that dear child walked into her room with a box of pizza and a movie, Mother was whisked away. Out of the wheelchair, out of the nursing home, out of the suffocating dementia.

Then, for the next couple of beautiful hours, Grandmother and Grandchild would sit, hand in hand, never letting go, and relish each other's company. Gram was content, she was safe, and she was happy. It was an oasis in the desert of dementia.

Dear Jesus, remind me that you hold my hand.
That you walk with me through this each week,
each day, and each hour. Thank you that with my
hand in yours, I am never alone.

Reflections:

_____

_____

_____

_____

_____

_____

JUNCTURE THIRTY-FIVE

He Knows My Name

"Listen to me, all of you in far-off lands: The Lord called me before my birth. From within the womb he called me by my name."
— (Isa. 49:1, TLB)

"The name of the Lord is a strong fortress; the godly run to him and are safe."
— (Prov. 18:10, NLT)

Names, dates, places, and events become noticeably unclear to the one suffering with dementia. As time progresses and the memories fade, these are lost one by one by one. To look at your parent—the one who raised you, nurtured you, taught you right from wrong, and most importantly guided you to the feet of Jesus—to look into their eyes and see vacant emptiness is extremely painful.

I remember the day vividly—Easter Sunday, April 4, 2010. It would be just five weeks later when Dad would receive perfect healing as he entered into eternity. By that Easter Day he was pretty much "gone" to us. He spent his days wandering around the locked wing of the nursing home or sitting, staring at the floor. He did not talk. He could do nothing for himself, not dressing, eating, nor bathing.

After our joyous church celebrations, a big Easter meal, and family traditions, my husband and I headed over to the nursing home to see Dad. It was dinner time. When we arrived a nurse was feeding him dinner, giving him bites of food as he opened his mouth for them, baby birdlike. I told her I would take over and she could help someone else. So, I sat down and began the honored task of gently nourishing the man who had raised me, loved me, protected me, and taught me about Jesus. My precious earthly father.

After a few uneventful spoonsful, I was given a glorious gift! My father, his head down, eyes unfocused on his plate of food, lost in Alzheimer's, SPOKE. And spoke clearly. He said, "Is that Joni right there?" He KNEW me! He knew ME! My dad, the one who sat with me in the night when I was a baby, who taught me to ride a bike, the one who consoled me when I failed my driving test, the one who walked me down the aisle on my wedding day—He KNEW my name! The name he had given me at birth. The name that identified me as his child. *Is that JONI right there?* Those were the last words I ever heard him say. It was incredible. It was enough.

How much more does our heavenly Father know us? How He loves us and protects us. He knew **our names** before we were born. And it is in **His Name** that we find our strength and protection.

Jesus, remind me to run to you, to know that your name is the name above all names. You are a strong tower, and in you I will find refuge.

Reflections:

_____
_____
_____
_____
_____

JUNCTURE THIRTY-SIX

God's Silent Witness

"Fixing our attention on Jesus, the pioneer and perfecter of the faith, who, in view of the joy set before him, endured the cross, disregarding its shame, and has sat down at the right hand of the throne of God."
— (HEB. 12:2, ISV)

It begins with forgetting seemingly inconsequential tidbits: where the socks are, what was for dinner, how to work the remote. It progresses: How do I get to the store? Did I pay that bill? Did we have lunch? And continues downward: I don't know how to get home, I don't know friends or family, I don't know how to bathe, dress, or eat.

In the latest stages of Alzheimer's, the words of Auguste Deter, the first person documented with the disease, ring true, "I have forgotten myself."

Thankfully, and mercifully, God has not forgotten. He is present, always.

Dad was weeks away from his eternal homegoing. He didn't know us, he couldn't speak, he spent his days roaming endlessly and aimlessly through the locked wing of the nursing facility.

We discovered he had begun a curious habit. The nurse on duty pulled us aside and informed us that there was a slight problem. Dad, in his meanderings, had been going into two particular residents' rooms—regularly—these same two rooms. He would sit on the bed and stare out of the window, again and again. Over and over. It was disconcerting since each of the rooms was occupied by a female. The ladies were becoming agitated with Dad frequenting their rooms, sitting on the bed, and gazing through the window.

The wonderful nurse said she had studied the two rooms, looked out and around the windows, and believed she knew the cause of Dad visiting the two rooms.

It was the CROSS. In both rooms, hanging in the window, was a cross. He was gazing at the CROSS. The CROSS was drawing him into those rooms. In the final stages of Alzheimer's, when he was unable to care for himself, to communicate, or recognize his loved ones, he knew where to go . . . to the CROSS. In the darkest recesses of the darkest disease, he was able to commune with the

One who transcends it all. He was in communion with his Savior, through the CROSS.

The nurse pulled me aside and asked if I thought we could hang a cross in Dad's room. Certainly, we could. Our youngest son, Lane, asked if he could make the cross to hang in his papa's room. He lovingly crafted it from two good-sized, rough logs. It was perfect.

Jesus, thank you for the beautifully poignant reminder to look to the cross. Thank you that you transcend even Alzheimer's.

Reflections:

_____

_____

_____

_____

_____

Forever Young

> *"I will declare that your love stands firm **forever**,*
> *that you have established your faithfulness in*
> *heaven itself."*
> — (Ps. 89:2, NIV)

No sense of reality. A dementia sufferer has little or no sense of reality. Their minds and eyes are clouded with the fog of unrealistic perceptions. These are sometimes alarming, sometimes sad, sometimes humorous, but always unrealistic.

By now, Mom was confined to a wheelchair. At age eighty with Alzheimer's, she was unable to dress herself, bathe herself, or walk more than a step or two. She didn't know what day, year, or season it was. She couldn't even turn on the television!

Dad had been gone nearly a year. Mom had been in a deep valley—we thought we were losing her—and soon. At Christmastime she was admitted to the hospital with pneumonia. Most folks in her condition don't recover. My brother had flown in to sit with us for these last days. Miraculously she woke up, she rallied, and improved tremendously! We were NOT prepared for what came next.

Mom said to my brother and me, "What do you kids think if I would remarry?" We were absolutely flabbergasted! After being shocked and speechless for a moment, I asked her if she had someone in mind. Well, yes. Actually, she did. *How interesting*. She began to describe this very nice young man she knew. He was going to be a doctor. He was kind, patient, and helpful. He came from a good family; his parents owned a farm nearby. I was trying to figure out how she met someone in her condition when I realized she was describing a young man in his twenties who was a CNA at the nursing home! He took care of her often, helping her walk, dress, eat, and get the TV on. In her Alzheimer's fog, she saw herself as a young woman needing the companionship and comfort of a husband.

My brother and I found it humorous and made some jokes with each other about borrowing the car keys from our new step-dad who was half our age! She had no idea of the utter impossibility of such a thing. The thought left her eventually—although there were two other men she considered eligible.

In my finite, realistic perception, this is a glimpse of heaven. We will spend eternity with no constraints of time, age, or illness. We will be forever young.

Jesus, thank you for a glimpse of heaven's reality
in Alzheimer's. Please continue to remind me that
your love stands firm forever.

<u>Reflections:</u>

_____

_____

_____

_____

_____

JUNCTURE THIRTY-EIGHT

This Kiss of Peace

> *"Love and faithfulness meet together; righteousness and peace kiss each other."*
> — (Ps. 85:10, NIV)

During the course of Alzheimer's, the days can become a series of incidents to navigate through. As the caregiver you plunge forward, solve the problems of the day, or the hour, or the moment, while managing your own life on the sidelines. It is constant pressure, expectations, demands, decisions, and it is emotionally and physically draining. Exhaustion is a frequent companion.

It was Sunday.

Sunday's were draining days. As the pastor's wife of a fairly good-sized church, I had some responsibilities— and definite expectations! I always sat in the front pew, supporting my husband and praying for him as God worked through him. I attempted to greet and visit with as many folks as possible during the back-to-back morning services. I checked on those who were having difficulties, I sympathized, and empathized. I prayed for folks. I loved on the babies and children. I checked on our staff's wives, and their families.

I was not only the pastor's wife, I was mother to three precious children in their late childhood, early teen years. I still had to get them up, get them going, make sure they were presentable, and ready to go on time. If they had money or forms due for an activity or trip, it seemed it was always Sunday morning when they remembered to tell us!

Sundays were beautiful, busy, and very tiring. It had been that way nearly my entire life. I had grown up in a home where it was an almost identical scenario, except my mom had four children to get ready and out the door!

It was Mother's Day Sunday. A day to celebrate, recognize, remember, and honor our mothers. The ones who carried us, fed us, bathed us, loved, rocked and kissed us. The women who prayed for us, cried for us, and hurt for us. Whether they were overbearing, or unassuming, they were ours.

My mother was confined by Alzheimer's in a nursing home, not understanding why I wouldn't take her to church, somehow always seeming to know when it was Sunday. She longed to go, but it was completely impossible at this stage.

I *wanted* to be with her, BUT . . .

It was Mother's Day! I was a mother—my children would come and surround me in the pew that morning! We would have a larger-than-average crowd that day. My husband would need me, the church folks would need me, the visitors would need me, the kids would need me, the wives, and babies would need me . . . I needed to be there.

I *wanted* to be with *my* mom, BUT so many people needed me . . .

Realizing what the future with Alzheimer's looked like, I decided to spend that Mother's Day Sunday morning with Mother. I didn't show up at church, I didn't sit with my children, I didn't love on all the folks. I went to the nursing home.

When I walked into her room, she looked up, and was so happy to see me. She knew me, she knew it was Sunday, she knew it was Mother's Day.

God blanketed us with a holy peace and calm that morning. We sensed His presence and enjoyed some special conversation, Scripture reading, and prayer. We admired the beautiful tree outside her window, as spring was bringing it to life. God sent His "kiss of peace" to both of us that day. It was beautiful and sublime.

It was the last Mother's Day I was to spend with my mother. I thought I was going to keep her company, that I magnanimously left my responsibilities for her. But I was wrong. Those amazing moments of God's peace and love that enveloped us were for me. I am undeservingly grateful.

Thank you, Jesus, for the meeting of your love and faithfulness—and the beautiful expression of your kiss of peace. Remind me that I always have access to that peace.

Reflections:

_____

_____

_____

_____

_____

JUNCTURE THIRTY-NINE

Inconspicuous Wealth

*"And my God will meet all your needs according to
the **riches** of his glory in Christ Jesus."*
— (PHIL. 4:19, NIV)

*". . . we ourselves are like fragile clay jars
containing this great **treasure**. This makes it clear
that our great power is from God,
not from ourselves."*
— (2 COR. 4:7, NLT)

Much of the journey through dementia is filled with confusion, misunderstanding, frustration, and unrecognizable actions. Watching a loved one fall further and further into the clutches of the disease is extremely difficult.

Walking the journey through dementia with a loved one and Jesus gives unimaginable strength, courage, and hope. And sometimes an unexpected example of grace and faithfulness.

Mom's last twenty-two months on Earth were spent in a nursing home. Spent in a nursing home, it was not fancy and was very institutionally functional. Gratefully, she was able to be in a room by herself. The room was approximately fifteen feet by ten feet. In this small living space was a standard issue hospital bed, her motorized lift chair from home, a dresser that she and Dad purchased their first year of marriage, a mini fridge, and a very small bathroom. Along with the couple of furniture pieces to try to make her feel "at home," we also brought some familiar pictures and hung them on the walls. That was it. A lifetime of decorating, arranging, appreciating, and welcoming guests in her home was boiled down to this one little room with a smattering of familiar items.

Each time I walked in the room, I was saddened by the situation. I was distressed that the vibrant, energetic, fruitful life my mother had lived had come to this existence, "languishing" in a nursing home. It weighed heavily on me. It was disheartening.

But Mom didn't see it that way. Mom saw it differently. When we would be there with her and someone walked in the room, she would say, "I am rich! Look at my family, God has blessed me. Look at my grandchildren who love me, God has blessed me. I am rich!" When one of my siblings from far away would call, she would hang up the phone and say, "I am rich! God has blessed me. My children love me, call me, and care about me. I am rich!" When visitors would come, old friends and new, she would say, "I am rich! God has blessed me. Just look at those who love me, I am rich!" When she saw a bird on the branch out the window, she would say, "I am rich to have this view of God's beautiful creation. I am rich!"

Mom understood about her riches, they were not in the temporal, her riches were not tied up in the depressing constraints the world had on her, but on the eternal. Not in things, but in those whom she poured her life into, for the sake of Christ. She taught me and my family a wonderful lesson during those twenty-two months. She was rich, and so can we be.

Thank you, Jesus, that in a seemingly discouraging and little nursing-home room, you showed us your inconspicuous wealth that is abundant and overflowing. Always. Thank you, Thank you.

Reflections:

_____

_____

_____

_____

_____

JUNCTURE FORTY

No Surprise

*"No one can deny it—God is really good to
Israel, and to all those with pure hearts. But I
nearly missed seeing it for myself."*
— (Ps. 73:1, TPT)

One of the markers of an individual suffering from dementia is the inability to perform everyday tasks. That statement may seem broad and vague, unless you are walking alongside someone who is exhibiting these inabilities. A myriad of "everyday tasks" become impossible, such as grooming, eating, or cooking, but a paramount one is the handling of money. At least for me it was.

My parents were "old school"—they didn't discuss their money with us kids. Dad was a savvy money manager and had an ample and comfortable retirement set up for him and Mom. He was very proud of that. Then Alzheimer's came to town. Alzheimer's that zaps logic and reasoning. Thankfully, and providentially, Dad gave me access and control of their finances. It was a monumental responsibility, and it was a crushing weight on me.

So many decisions, so many voices vying for input on what to do. My ultimate objective was to honor my parents and provide the finest care. It was frightening to watch the bank account drain like a sieve each month that both of them were living in a nursing facility.

I worried consistently and chronically about it. I knew there were laws and regulations about what could and couldn't be done, and I didn't want to jeopardize their quality of care, or my legal status. My paramount concern was what would happen when it ran out. I knew they would have to go on government assistance. I know it happens every day. I just did not want that to be the final chapter in my folks' life. For their sake. For my sake. I couldn't stomach the thought. But it was coming, and it was inevitable. Every month when I wrote the check for the nursing home, it was becoming imminent. Every month the end of the money was drawing nearer. Every month I was sinking deeper into despair over the situation. Every month seemed to roll around much too quickly.

Becky was the financial administrator of the nursing home. A sweet, pleasant, and cheerful person, I visited with her each month when I went in to pay my parents' bill. I shared my trepidation and anxiety about the upcoming deficit. She was quick to assure me that she would help walk me through the process, when it was time. That gave me a bit of comfort. Becky said to let her know when the bank account was at two thousand dollars—that was when we had to act. I assured her I would.

It was December. The "most wonderful time of the year"—not so for me. I was distraught to realize that the fateful two-thousand-dollar mark had arrived. I knew I had to call Becky. I put it off for days. I had a lump in my throat and a knot in my stomach. I was terrified. No matter what happened, it was all on my shoulders, I was legally responsible. Finally, I took a deep breath, picked up the phone, and I called.

When I explained to Becky that the time had come, we were done, out of money, needing to sign up for government assistance, she gave me an amazingly profound response.

Her simple, seven-word reply, "THIS is NOT a surprise to God."

THIS terrible, awful, sickening situation I had fretted, worried, and despaired over, THIS, is NOT a surprise for MY God! Somewhere along the way I had pushed that knowledge aside. Somehow, I thought I had to take care of it. At some point I had taken hold of the reigns. I thought I had to take care of it.

Becky was God's messenger that day. With indescribable relief, I thanked her, hung up the phone, and cried like a baby! All the while thanking and praising our glorious God and Savior who sent Becky along to remind me WHO was in control, who was with me all along, and who would continue to be on this next phase of the journey!

Those words are with me daily, "THIS is NOT a surprise to God."

Jesus, I exalt you! Thank you for the reminder that **nothing** *can surprise you. You have been, and always will be, there for us as we look to you for guidance.*

Reflections:

_____

_____

_____

_____

_____

JUNCTURE FORTY-ONE

Not Just Some Things, but All

*"(For) we know that all things work together for good to those who love God, to those who are the called according to **His** purpose."*
— (ROM. 8:28, MEV)

Walking alongside someone with dementia/Alzheimer's may be the hardest task you ever face. It was for me. As the disease progressed, it became a downward spiral, as Dad, then Mom, progressively worsened. Each day held an uncertain dread. I didn't see how any of it could be working out for good—it all felt bad to me.

It was then, at my lowest and darkest, while Mom was very close to entering eternity, that I was reminded.

Romans 8:28 was Mom's life verse. She had lived quite a life. Romans 8:28 was her verse after surviving a tornado and losing everything she owned. Through the sickness and death of a husband, she claimed Romans 8:28. As a single mom, Romans 8:28 sustained her. Marrying Dad, and through ministry literally from coast to coast, she was adamant that Romans 8:28 was true.

From my earliest memories, as she tucked me in at night, the last thing I remember hearing her say was, "For we know that ALL things work together for good . . ."

As my sister and I sat by her nursing-home bedside, she was virtually unresponsive, slipping from this life to eternity, and we witnessed an amazing event. One after another residents, residents' families, nurses, aides, administrators, kitchen staff, housekeeping, maintenance, and transportation came to visit. Each one had a special memory, moment, or ritual that they shared uniquely with mom. Each one would lean over, remind her of the situation, give a praise report, and express their love and gratitude. She would respond in a deep, raspy voice, "I love you." It was overwhelming. She gave the hope of Jesus and a little piece of herself to everyone who crossed her path. In the nursing home, in one tiny, stifling room. In the ugly, sticky, miry confusion of Alzheimer's. Romans 8:28. When I thought she was languishing the last two years, she was showing Jesus, as she had always done. She knew God would ALWAYS work everything out, and she didn't stop trusting Him. It was that simple.

God sent me a message that weekend. One I already knew but had let the weight of my humanness creep in and push it aside.

Romans 8:28—ALL things work together for good.

Thank you, Jesus, for always being there.
Please help us never forget you are always working
on our behalf as we trust in you.

<u>Reflections:</u>

_____

_____

_____

_____

_____

JUNCTURE FORTY-TWO

Beautiful Butterfly

*"But let me reveal to you a wonderful secret. We
will not all die, but we will all be transformed."*
— (1 COR. 15:51, NLT)

For someone suffering with Alzheimer's disease, there
may be a point of reference that loved ones or caregivers
can use in communication.

Butterflies. On the walls, paintings, prints, and drawn
by amateurs. Quilts, pillows, and rugs. Butterflies. On
dishes, cups, towels, and ephemera. On clothing, on lamps,
on clocks, and furniture. Butterflies. They were *everywhere*!
She didn't just *love* butterflies, she was immersed in and
consumed by them. She was a butterfly junkie. And everyone
knew it—the church folk, the kids in her classroom, the
parents of the kids in her classroom, the teachers she worked
with, her friends at the Y, her friends at the beauty shop, her

friends at the grocery store. Her family. We all knew about the butterflies.

It was the brooches, or for simplicity, pins. The butterfly pins given and collected over a lifetime that gave evidence of her soaring spirit. Every day, for approximately forty years, when she arrived at school, she was wearing a butterfly pin. Oh, but Mrs. McCleery of the aptly named "McCleery's Monarchs" class wouldn't just be wearing a pin every day on her lapel. No, no, no. The pin was strategically placed as though it had just gently landed. Sometimes on her shoulder, sometimes on her wrist, or elbow, or her hair, or her back. The children would eagerly anticipate her arrival each day to discover the latest landing! Enchanting.

She loved their beauty, colors, and their gentle strength. She loved their story. The transformational story of the butterfly was Joan McCleery. She understood. She was captivated. It was her story. The butterfly was always about new life, from the Life Giver Himself, Jesus. And on a cold day in January a few years ago, she shed her worldly, sickly, and confused confines. She flew from this world and landed safely and gently in her Savior's arms.

I praise you, Lord, for your transforming power.
Please remind me often.

Reflections:

_____

_____

_____

_____

_____

JUNCTURE FORTY-THREE

Run to Jesus

*"The name of the Lord is a strong fortress; the godly
run to him and are safe. "*
— (PROV. 18:10, NLT)

Watching a loved one descend into Alzheimer's evokes many unusual and fascinating paradigm shifts. The person afflicted can act in new, different, and uncharacteristic ways. Or you will glimpse their "normal" character, raw and exposed, without the filters of propriety guiding them.

My mother was married at age seventeen. Just a child in love with a war veteran. He was an older, handsome, Navy man, stationed on the USS Missouri and actually witnessed the signing of the treaty to end World War II—"Unconditional Surrender." Pretty impressive! More than that, he was called to preach! He was bold, charismatic, and ready to win the world for Jesus!

What my mother didn't know, until after they were married, is that he was sick. While in the war, he had contracted jungle fever, a severe form of malaria, which weakened his heart. And after ten years of marriage and much sickness, he passed away leaving my mother a widow with two young children at age twenty-seven.

God, in his great providence brought my father along to marry my mother and adopt the two children as his own—and two more children came along a few years later. He, too, was a minister, and they had a wonderful, fruitful ministry together.

Fast forward fifty years. My father had passed away. Mother had now outlived two husbands. She was completely distraught, despondent, sinking, and suffering from Alzheimer's. We feared she was going to follow my father to heaven very shortly. Then something fascinating happened. She perked up a bit. She rallied. And she became fixated on a single thought that absolutely, wholeheartedly consumed her.

"I have TWO husbands in heaven—what am I going to do when I get there? Who do I run to first?"

She asked this question of everyone she came in contact with. Every one. The nurses, the staff, other residents, visitors, my siblings, my children, my husband, and me. "What am I going to do when I get to heaven? I have TWO husbands there. Who do I run to first?" Over and over, she asked "the question."

Some people were uncomfortable, and some people were baffled. Many folks told us she had asked them "the question" and they didn't know how to respond.

But my husband, Doug, had no trouble knowing the perfect answer. Every time she asked him (and she asked him countless times), "What am I going to do when I get to heaven?" He would respond, "Just run to Jesus, and everything else will work out." Oh, that makes sense. "Yes, just run to Jesus and everything else will work out." That simple, yet profound answer would satisfy her . . . until she forgot and asked again, and again, and again.

"Just run to Jesus, and everything else will work out."

"Just run to Jesus . . ."

Dear Jesus, help us remember that you are the consummate answer to all our questions. We can "just run to you." Thank you.

Reflections:

_____

_____

_____

_____

_____

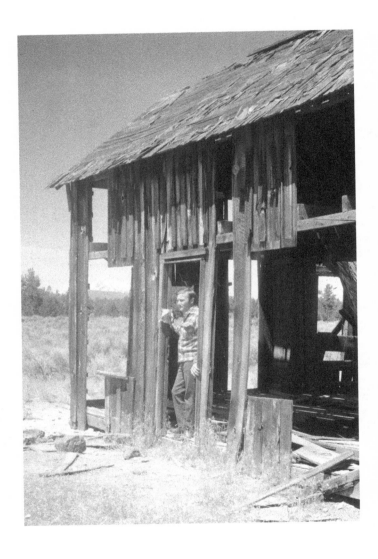

JUNCTURE FORTY-FOUR

Faithful Feet

*"He will guard the **feet** of his faithful servants."*
— (1 SAM. 2:9, NIV)

*"How beautiful on the mountains are the feet of
the messenger who brings good news, the good news
of peace and salvation, the news that the God of
Israel reigns!"*
— (ISA. 52:7, NLT)

When you know nothing about something, it's unnerving.

In the mid 1970s, my mother had an operation. She was going to be spending several days in the hospital. My father allowed me to miss a day of high school to stay with my mom in her hospital room. I did not enjoy that day. At all. That was the day I knew unequivocally I was not wired for any kind of career in the medical field! That still holds true today. God called me to be a teacher, and he called others to work in medicine.

One such person was Amy. Through the Alzheimer's journey with both of my parents, I was very grateful for all the kind, helpful, and knowledgeable medical personnel who cared for them.

But then there was Amy.

Amy showed up toward the end. She was a nurse in the last facility. She cared for my parents as though they were her own. Amy made me feel as though my parents were the most important ones in her care. Amy called the doctor when she thought meds should be adjusted. She was gentle, kind, and confident. Amy told me I needed to take care of myself. Amy looked out for visitors who came to visit. She was an incredible gift to me and my family.

During the unending days of Alzheimer's, my husband, Doug, and I were supposed to fly to Florida for a short getaway. Dad was declining rapidly, and I was afraid to leave. I thought we should scrap the trip. I would have been devastated if he slipped into eternity while we were gone. Amy told me she wanted to show me something and took me to the end of Dad's bed. She pulled the sheets up and said, "Look at his feet." I looked. I saw an elderly man's feet. The feet of a "faithful servant." Feet of a "messenger who had shared the Good News of salvation." They looked old, sick, and tired to me. Amy explained that what she saw were feet that weren't ready to leave this world yet. She knew the signs—Dad's feet were still on this side of eternity. We could leave and be confident he would still be with us when we got back. I trusted Amy, so we left. She was right about his feet. Dad was still with us for several more weeks.

For my family, for my parents, Amy was the one with, "beautiful feet." She was the tireless messenger, giving us hope, help, care, encouragement—and reality—when we needed it.

When I read Isaiah 52:7, "How beautiful on the mountains are the feet of the messenger" . . . I think not of Amy, the nurse. But Amy, my friend.

Jesus, I praise you for your wonderful gift of Amy.
Thank you for someone with beautiful feet to walk
us through the dark days. I pray you gift an "Amy"
to all on this difficult path.

Reflections:

_____

_____

_____

_____

_____

TEN DO'S AND DON'TS FOR ALZHEIMER'S CAREGIVERS

1. Don't be in denial. Be proactive. It's natural to be in denial when a loved one begins to show signs of dementia, but that prevents the person from getting a diagnosis, starting treatment, and planning for the future.

2. Don't ask, "Do you remember?" Be mindful of how you say things. No, they don't remember. Asking if they remember some person or event could make them frustrated and upset.

3. Do interact with the person at their level. Join their reality. You may want to interact with the person the way you always have, but that isn't going to be possible. Instead, figure out the level at which they are behaving and connect on that level.

4. Do use touch, sights, sounds, smells and taste as forms of communication. Smile, hold hands, play their favorite music. Bring children, or pets. It's not all about words.

5. Do know when you need a moment. Sometimes it helps to "reset." Step outside for a moment or go to a different room. Close your eyes and take a couple of deep breaths. You don't want any regrets.

6. Don't argue, correct, or disagree. You can't win an argument with a person who has dementia. Neither should you contradict them. It will make them, and you, both frustrated.

7. Do look for the underlying emotion in what is being communicated. Attend to the emotion. If your loved one keeps saying that they "want to go home," they may be feeling unsafe or insecure. Try reassuring the person and redirecting the conversation or activity.

8. Do quickly change the subject if the person gets upset. If the person gets upset, one of the best things you can do is redirect their attention to something else. It may help to take the blame, even if it's not your fault. Is it more helpful to be right or to be kind?

9. Don't quit visiting when the person doesn't know who you are. Just because your loved one does not recognize you doesn't mean that you will not benefit from seeing them.

10. Do take care of yourself. Being an Alzheimer's caregiver is exhausting work. Take good care of yourself for your benefit and for the good of the person for whom you're caring. You can't be an effective, compassionate caregiver if you're weary and burned out all the time.

SOME HELPFUL RESOURCES

Alzheimer's Caregiving | National Institute on Aging
https://www.nia.nih.gov/health/alzheimers/caregiving

Tips for Alzheimer's Caregivers: Preparing for the Road Ahead
https://www.helpguide.org/articles/alzheimers-dementia-aging/tips-for-alzheimers-caregivers.htm

Tips for Daily Life | Alzheimer's Association
https://www.alz.org/i-have-alz/tips-for-daily-life.asp

Caregiver's Guide to Understanding Dementia Behaviors
https://www.caregiver.org/caregivers-guide-understanding-dementia-behaviors

Alzheimer's Symptoms: 24 Signs & Symptoms of Alzheimer's Disease
https://www.webmd.com/alzheimers/guide/understanding-alzheimers-disease-symptoms

Alzheimer's Disease Symptoms & Signs | BrightFocus Foundation
https://www.brightfocus.org/alzheimers/symptoms-and-stages